Pediatric
health
case studies

Pediatric health case studies

Beverly R. Rothfeld, RN, MSN, CPNP
Special Assistant Professor
Graduate Nursing
Simmons College
Boston, Massachusetts
Pediatric Nurse Practitioner
Harvard Vanguard Medical Associates
West Roxbury, Massachusetts

Deborah A. Krepcio, RN-CS, MSN, CPNP
Pediatric Nurse Practitioner
Harvard Vanguard Medical Associates
Wellesley, Massachusetts
Adjunct Clinical Instructor
Graduate Nursing
Simmons College
Boston, Massachusetts

Appleton & Lange
Stamford, Connecticut

Copyright © 1999 by Appleton & Lange
A Simon & Schuster Company

www.appletonlange.com

99 00 01 02 / 11 10 9 8 7 6 5 4 3 2 1

Prentice Hall International (UK) Limited, *London*
Prentice Hall of Australia Pty. Limited, *Sydney*
Prentice Hall Canada, Inc., *Toronto*
Prentice Hall Hispanoamericana, S.A., *Mexico*
Prentice Hall of India Private Limited, *New Delhi*
Prentice Hall of Japan, Inc., *Tokyo*
Simon & Schuster Asia Pte. Ltd., *Singapore*
Editora Prentice Hall do Brasil Ltda., *Rio de Janeiro*
Prentice Hall, *Upper Saddle River, New Jersey*

Library of Congress Cataloging-in-Publication Data

Rothfeld, Beverly R.
    Pediatric health case studies / Beverly R. Rothfeld, Deborah A. Krepcio.
        p.   cm. — (Nurse practitioner certification review series)
    Includes bibliographical references.
    ISBN 0-8385-8137-4 (pbk. : alk. paper)
    1. Pediatric nursing—Examinations, questions, etc.   2. Nurse
practitioners—Examinations, questions, etc.   3. Nurse
practitioners—Certification.   I. Krepcio, Deborah A.   II. Title.
III. Series.
    [DNLM: 1. Pediatric Nursing examination questions.
2. Certification examination questions.   3. Nurse Practitioners
examination questions.   WY 18.2 R846p 1999]
RJ245.R68   1999
610.73'62'076—dc21
DNLM/DLC
for Library of Congress   98-22075
                                                                              CIP

Editor-in-Chief: Sally J. Barhydt
Production: Andover Publishing Services

ISBN 0-8385-8137-4

90000

9 780838 581377

PRINTED IN THE UNITED STATES OF AMERICA

Contents

Contributors

Mary Galvin, RN, MS, CPNP
Allied Pediatrics
West Bridgewater, Massachusetts

Robert A. Hoch, MD, MPH
Pediatrician and Medical Director
Neponset Health Center
Director of Pediatrics
Carney Hospital
Dorchester, Massachusetts

Patricia R. Lawrence, RN, MS, PNP
Boston Medical Center and Boston University
    School of Medicine
Boston, Massachusetts

Annie Lewis-O'Connor, MSN, MPH
Pediatric & Obstetric/Gynecologic Nurse
    Practitioner
Neponset Health Center
Dorchester, Massachusetts
Boston University School of Public Health
Boston, Massachusetts

Preface

This book has been developed for pediatric nurse practitioners who are preparing to take either the *National Qualifying Examination for Pediatric Nurse Practitioners* offered by The National Certification Board of Pediatric Nurse Practitioners and Nurses (NCBPNP/N) or the *Pediatric Nurse Practitioner Examination* offered by the American Nurses Credentialing Center (ANCC). Certification is important to nurse practitioners both as a means of maintaining high professional standards and as a vehicle for the establishment of the nurse practitioner role within the ever-evolving health care system. The objective of this book is to provide a self-study reference for entry-level pediatric nurse practitioners preparing for these examinations. The book can help determine the level of overall competence in pediatrics as well as identify specific content areas needing additional study.

This review book uses a case study format and contains over 500 test questions covering the content that you are most likely to encounter in the pediatric certification examinations. The case study format is intended to give the pediatric nurse practitioner an introduction to the examination process in a realistic practitioner–client setting. The case studies and test questions are designed to cover the general content areas of both examinations: health care delivery systems and methods, growth and development, health promotion, health maintenance, health restoration, and common acute and chronic clinical problems and illnesses. The correct answer and, more importantly, the rationale for the correct answer are also included. Some rationales provide necessary general information peripherally related to the subject matter of the individual case study in the form of tables or figures. References and additional bibliographical information can be found at the end of the book, grouped by subject area.

As certified pediatric nurse practitioners and graduate faculty, we recognize the need for a nurse practitioner certification examination review series that uses a case study approach. Our hope is that this format will help you gain the confidence needed to prepare for and successfully complete the certification process. We welcome your feedback on content and format, which will ultimately help us to improve our future efforts.

ACKNOWLEDGMENTS

A project such as this takes the encouragement and cooperation of a number of people. Our sincere appreciation goes to our editor and all the staff at Appleton & Lange, who not only made this book possible but made the process pleasurable. Thanks also to Niels Buessem at Andover Publishing Services for his expert support.

We also wish to thank our contributors for sharing their expertise:

Mary Galvin, CPNP—Professional Issues
Robert Hoch, MD—Gastrointestinal Disorders
Patricia Lawrence, CPNP—Pediatric Cardiology
Annie Lewis-O'Connor, MSN—Gynecology

Also, our sincere thanks to our students, colleagues, and friends who have offered suggestions and insight.

Most importantly, we would like to thank our families: Van, Sam, and Ellie; Bob, Beka, Ariel and Molly, and Mom and Dad, for their never-ending support and patience.

Beverly R. Rothfeld, RN, MSN, CPNP
Deborah A. Krepcio, RNCS, MSN, CPNP

About the Pediatric Nurse Practitioner Certification Exam

Two certification boards—the National Certification Board of Pediatric Nurse Practitioners and Nurses (NCBPNP/N) and the American Nurses Credentialing Center (ANCC)—offer certification examinations for qualified pediatric nurse practitioner candidates. Each of these examinations evaluates the pediatric nurse practitioner's entry-level knowledge and application of knowledge in the delivery of health care to children and families. It is the personal preference of the exam candidate that determines which examination is taken for certification.

NATIONAL QUALIFYING EXAMINATION FOR PEDIATRIC NURSE PRACTITIONERS

The National Qualifying Examination for Pediatric Nurse Practitioners is offered by the National Certification Board of Pediatric Nurse Practitioners and Nurses (NCBPNP/N). The examination consists of 200 multiple-choice questions in a computerized format. The test questions are designed to test the pediatric nurse practitioner's entry-level knowledge in the following areas: health care delivery–systems and methods, growth and development, health maintenance, and common clinical problems. The examination is offered three times a year and is administered at a Sylvan Technology Center. The candidate chooses one test date from a predesignated 12-day examina-

tion period. The predesignated examination periods for 1998 occur in March, August, and November. For 1999, the examination dates are February 22 to March 5, June 21 to July 2, and October 25 to November 5. The application process takes 4 to 8 weeks. On receipt of your application, NCBPNP/N will send you an examination description packet that includes an examination time schedule, letter of eligibility, directions for scheduling a test site and time, exam regulations, sample questions for practice, description of the scoring process, and a detailed content outline. Written notification of exam scores is sent directly to each candidate within 6 weeks after the last test date of the 12-day exam period. The 1998 fee for certification is $350.00, which includes a $250.00 exam fee and a $100.00 nonrefundable registration fee. Certification remains active for 6 years and is maintained through a certification maintenance program that includes yearly self-assessment learning exercises and continuing education credit (CEU) documentation. The certification maintenance program is outlined in the information booklet provided with the examination application.

To obtain an application and information booklet, contact the National Certification Board of Pediatric Nurse Practitioners and Nurses, 800 South Frederick Avenue, Suite 104, Gaithersburg, MD 20877-4150, (888-641-2767). You may also obtain an application and information through the NCBPNP/N internet site (http://www.pnpcert.org).

PEDIATRIC NURSE PRACTITIONER EXAMINATION

The Pediatric Nurse Practitioner Examination is offered by the American Nurses Credentialing Center (ANCC). The examination consists of multiple-choice questions in a paper-and-pencil format. The test questions are designed to test the pediatric nurse practitioner's entry-level knowledge in the following areas: health promotion, health maintenance, health restoration, acute illnesses, chronic diseases, and disabilities. The examination is offered three times a year and is administered at various test sites throughout the United States over a one-day examination period. The one-day examination periods for 1998 occur in February, June, and October. In 1999, the first examination date is February 6, with additional examinations in June and October. On receipt of your application, ANCC will send you an information guide to the examination that contains information about the exam process, test content outline, exam site, admission ticket, and sample test questions. Written notification of exam scores is sent directly to each candidate within 6 to 8 weeks after the exam date. The 1998 fee for certification is $296.00, with a discounted rate of $156.00 for those qualifying individuals who have been members of the American Nurses Association or their State Nurses Association for at least 6 months prior to the application date. Certification remains active for 5 years and is maintained by meeting the practice requirements as specified in your area of certification and by obtaining yearly continuing education credits (CEUs). The requirements for recertification are sent to you with your certificate and are available in the ANCCs recertification catalog.

To obtain an application and information catalog, contact the American Nurses Credentialing Center, 600 Maryland Avenue SW, Suite 100 West, Washington, DC, 20024-2571, (800) 284-2378. You may also obtain a catalog and application through the American Nurses Association internet site (http://www.nursingworld.org).

I

Health Maintenance and Promotion

Cases and Questions

HISTORY TAKING AND PHYSICAL EXAMINATION

1. Which of the following communication techniques would be *most* helpful in taking a history of a child who is in respiratory distress from an asthma attack?

   (A) Open-ended questions
   (B) Nonverbal communication
   (C) Close-ended questions
   (D) Pauses and silent periods

2. Which of the following communication techniques would be *most* helpful when speaking to a parent who has had a recent loss in the family?

   (A) Clarification
   (B) Summarizing information
   (C) Close-ended questions
   (D) Empathy

3. An effective interview with an adolescent client requires an Advanced Practice Nurse to

   (A) Use a lot of current teenage vernacular
   (B) Get the sensitive topics out of the way early on
   (C) Recognize the adolescent's positive attributes
   (D) Include the parent in all encounters with the adolescent

4. Essential elements of interviewing patients include all the following EXCEPT

   (A) Informed consent
   (B) Assurance of privacy and confidentiality
   (C) Minimum interruptions
   (D) Detailed note taking

5. The communication approach that is *most* helpful when bringing up sensitive issues is known as

   (A) The depersonalized question
   (B) The direct question
   (C) The confrontational question
   (D) The close-ended question

6. An example of an open-ended question is

   (A) Do you get headaches?
   (B) How are things at home?
   (C) Have you had sore throats?
   (D) Have you ever been hospitalized?

7. Clarification as a communication technique may be helpful when information is

   (A) Comical
   (B) Insensitive
   (C) Confusing
   (D) Personal

8. Which of the following is/are (a) potential barrier(s) to effective communication?

   (A) Cultural differences
   (B) Frequent interruptions
   (C) Lack of continuity of care
   (D) All of the above

9. Of the following, which is *not* usually indicated in a history of a child acutely ill with pharyngitis?

    (A) History of present illness (HPI)
    (B) Review of systems (ROS)
    (C) Genogram
    (D) Chief complaint

10. A new mother presents at the 2-week visit with her newborn. She appears tired and teary and states that she wishes she never had a baby. What is an appropriate response?

    (A) "Your baby is so cute. How can you say that?"
    (B) "You sound like you are feeling overwhelmed."
    (C) "Oh come on. It can't be that bad."
    (D) "I know a lot of people who would love to have a baby."

11. A suggested order of the physical exam in young children is

    (A) Heart, lungs, abdomen
    (B) Ears, oropharynx, genitalia
    (C) Genitalia, abdomen, skin
    (D) None of the above

12. In a situation where a young child is resisting a physical exam, the most appropriate remark to the child would be

    (A) "If you don't hold still, I'll have to give you a shot."
    (B) "Why can't you be as good as my other patients are?"
    (C) "Why are you acting like a baby?"
    (D) "I can tell you're upset. Why do you feel so afraid today?"

13. A physical exam of a fearful 2-year-old should be done

    (A) On the exam table
    (B) On the parent's lap
    (C) With the parent out of the room
    (D) With the child restrained

14. The physical exam of the prepubescent child is best accomplished

    (A) With attention to modesty issues
    (B) With clothes left on
    (C) With the parent in attendance
    (D) With the siblings in the exam room

15. Expected percussion findings over a healthy liver are

    (A) Resonant
    (B) Hyperresonant
    (C) Tympanic
    (D) Dull

16. Normal percussion findings over a hyperinflated area are

    (A) Hyperresonant
    (B) Dull
    (C) Tympanic
    (D) Flat

17. Bruits can be an abnormal finding on a physical exam and are found during

    (A) Inspection
    (B) Auscultation
    (C) Percussion
    (D) Palpation

18. Crackles are findings often heard with which of these conditions?

    (A) Hyperactive peristalsis
    (B) Pneumonia
    (C) Congenital hip dysplasia (CHD)
    (D) Nonfunctional murmurs

19. The Romberg test examines which of the following functions?

    (A) Peripheral vascular system
    (B) Auditory system
    (C) Cerebellar system
    (D) Respiratory system

20. A normal Rinne test demonstrates which of the following?

(A) Intact cranial nerve VIII
(B) Intact cranial nerves IX and X
(C) Intact cranial nerve XI
(D) Intact cranial nerve XII

IMMUNIZATIONS

Questions 21–23

Stephen is a full-term, healthy male infant here today with his parent for a 2-month health supervision visit. An important part of his visit today will be administration of several immunizations. He has previously received two doses of hepatitis B virus vaccine without adverse reaction.

21. Which of the following statements, noted during today's interview, will determine the type of polio vaccine that Stephen will receive?

    (A) This child currently has a monilial diaper dermatitis.
    (B) He is breast-fed.
    (C) His 3-year-old sibling currently has an upper respiratory infection with low-grade fever.
    (D) His paternal grandmother, who resides in the household, is receiving chemotherapy for colon cancer.

22. According to the 1997 Immunization Guidelines, which of the following polio vaccine regimes should Stephen receive?

    (A) OPV only at 2, 4, and 6–18 months and at 4–6 years
    (B) IPV at 2 and 4 months, OPV at 12–18 months and at 4–6 years
    (C) IPV only at 2, 4, and 12–18 months and at 4–6 years
    (D) None of the above

23. Each of the three vaccine schedules (IPV only, OPV only, OPV–IPV) are highly effective. Major factors for the PNP in the selection of the most appropriate polio vaccine option include

    (A) Parent and/or provider choice
    (B) Risk of vaccine-associated paralytic poliomyelitis (VAPP)
    (C) Number of injections required at scheduled visits to administer recommended vaccines
    (D) All of the above

Questions 24–26

John is a 5-year-old boy with a past medical history of moderate asthma. His asthma at present is under excellent control. His daily asthma meds consist of cromolyn sodium (Intal) two puffs tid and albuterol (Ventolin) two puffs tid. His last episode of asthma that required a short burst of corticosteroids (1–2 mg/kg) was 8 months ago.

24. In addition to receiving those immunizations recommended in the current guidelines for pediatric immunizations, which of the following immunizations would you recommend for John based on his history of moderate asthma?

    1. Pneumococcal vaccine
    2. Influenza vaccine

    (A) 1 only
    (B) 2 only
    (C) 1 and 2
    (D) Neither vaccine is recommended.

25. Which of the following children would you recommend receive influenza immunization?

    (A) A healthy 12-month-old who attends day care regularly
    (B) A 12-month-old child with sickle cell anemia
    (C) A 17-year-old sexually active teenager
    (D) All of the above

26. Which of the following children should receive pneumococcal immunization?

    (A) A 12-month-old who has a history of frequent otitis media
    (B) A 4-year-old with HIV
    (C) A 15-year-old with a history of moderate asthma
    (D) All of the above

Questions 27–33

Marie-Louise, a 6-year-old child from Haiti, and her 11-year-old brother, Michel, recently joined their family living in the United States. They are here today for routine health supervision. They are both healthy, with no previous history of significant illness or hospitalization. They will attend a local public school, and their immunization status is unknown. The physical examination and developmental screening are normal for both children.

27. According to the current recommendations, which of the following immunizations would Marie-Louise need to receive at this first visit for school entry in the fall?

    1. DTaP
    2. Hib
    3. HBV
    4. Polio
    5. MMR

    (A) 1, 3, 4, and 5
    (B) 1, 2, and 4
    (C) 1 and 4
    (D) All of the above

28. Michel is unable to receive all needed vaccines simultaneously. Which would be the most important for him to receive at today's visit?

    (A) DTaP
    (B) Polio
    (C) MMR
    (D) Hib

29. Which of the following is a contraindication to receiving MMR vaccine?

    (A) Asymptomatic HIV infection
    (B) Pregnancy
    (C) Upper respiratory infection with temperature <37.7°C (100°F)
    (D) All of the above

30. Common presenting signs and symptoms of measles include

    (A) Dysphagia, conjunctivitis, fever
    (B) Morbilliform rash which begins on the torso
    (C) Conjunctivitis, coryza, cough
    (D) Headache, abdominal pain, exudative pharyngitis

31. Rubella is characterized by all of the following EXCEPT

    (A) Generalized maculopapular rash which begins on the face and neck
    (B) Cervical lymphadenopathy
    (C) Koplik spots
    (D) Low-grade fever

32. Complications of mumps include all of the following EXCEPT

    (A) Orchitis
    (B) Pancreatitis
    (C) Meningitis
    (D) Pneumonia

33. Which of the following is a live vaccine?

    (A) IPV
    (B) Hepatitis B
    (C) MMR
    (D) DTaP

Questions 34–39

Jessie is a healthy infant who presents today for a 4-month well-child visit. She is currently up to date with all recommended health supervision visits and immunizations. She has had no adverse reaction to previous immunizations and has no known allergies. She is currently well and afebrile and has had no recent illnesses, injuries, or hospitalizations.

34. Which of the following immunizations will be administered to Jessie at today's 4-month health supervision visit?

    (A) DTaP, Hib
    (B) DTaP, Hib, polio
    (C) DT, Hib
    (D) DT, Hib, polio

35. Prior to administrating the immunizations to Jessie, the PNP should

(A) Obtain informed consent, in writing, from the parent/guardian
(B) Provide a parent/guardian with a copy of the vaccine information statement prepared by the Centers for Disease Control (CDC)
(C) Provide the parent/guardian with every opportunity to ask questions and have those questions answered
(D) All of the above

36. Later that afternoon, Jessie's parent calls to report that Jessie has been irritable for several hours and has now developed a rectal temperature of 38.3°C (101°F). What would be the appropriate course of action regarding DTaP administration at this child's 6-month health supervision visit?

(A) Defer all immunizations until the child is 12 months of age.
(B) Defer immunization with the pertussis vaccine and, instead, administer diphtheria and tetanus toxoid vaccine (DT).
(C) Administer half the usual dose of the DTaP vaccine.
(D) Administer the DTaP vaccine with instructions for fever control.

37. The most common adverse reaction to DTaP immunization is

(A) Fever of 40.0°C (104°F) or greater
(B) Local pain and swelling at the injection site
(C) Prolonged crying
(D) Irritability

38. The most appropriate advice the PNP could offer regarding this child's postimmunization reaction is

(A) Review common postimmunization reactions and tell the parent to administer acetaminophen (15 mg/kg/dose) every 4 hours as needed for pain and fever.
(B) Advise immediate appointment with the infant's primary care provider.
(C) Advise immediate hospital referral.
(D) None of the above.

39. Before the introduction of an effective vaccine, which of the following organisms was the most common cause of meningitis and epiglottitis in infants and young children?

(A) *Bordetella pertussis*
(B) *Haemophilis influenzae*
(C) *Streptococcus pneumoniae*
(D) Measles virus

Questions 40–46

Joelle is a 5-hour-old, healthy, full-term female infant born to a healthy gravida 2, para 2 mother who had a healthy pregnancy and uncomplicated vaginal delivery. Joelle's mother was prenatally tested for hepatitis B and was found to be HBsAg negative.

40. Joelle should receive her *initial dose* of hepatitis B vaccine

(A) In 1 month
(B) Within the first 12 hours after birth
(C) In 6 months
(D) Within the first 12 hours after birth along with hepatitis B immune globulin (HBIG)

At Joelle's 2-week health supervision visit, her mother has questions regarding hepatitis B vaccination for her previously unvaccinated 12-year-old son. He has no known risk factors for HBV infection or family members with active or chronic HBV infection.

41. Based on the currently 1997 guidelines for childhood immunization and knowledge of HBV transmission, what would your recommendation be for pre-exposure HBV immunization for this 12-year-old?

(A) Since he is not at high risk for HBV, no vaccination is recommended at this time.
(B) All children who have not been previously immunized by or before age 11–12 years should receive HBV vaccine.
(C) HBV immunization is recommended upon entrance to college.
(D) None of the above.

42. Prior to administration of the HBV vaccine, this 12-year-old's parent reports that the child has had a mild URI with low-grade fever and a dry cough. In light of his recent mild URI, the PNP should

    (A) Defer administration of HBV vaccine until the child is entirely well as URI with low-grade fever is a true contra-indication to vaccine administration.
    (B) Administer the HBV vaccine at today's visit because URI with low-grade fever is not a true contraindication to vaccine administration.
    (C) Defer vaccine administration for 6 months.
    (D) This child is not a candidate to receive HBV vaccine.

43. Which of the following is true about hepatitis B?

    (A) The incubation period is 2–6 months.
    (B) Breast-feeding by an HBsAg-positive mother is contraindicated.
    (C) The vaccine for hepatitis B carries a minimal risk of HIV infection.
    (D) Ingestion of contaminated food or water is the most common mode of transmission.

44. All of the following statements regarding hepatitis A are true EXCEPT

    (A) It has an abrupt onset.
    (B) Transmission is primarily through sexual contract.
    (C) Chronic hepatitis does not occur post-infection.
    (D) HAV is highly contagious.

45. The hepatitis virus that is responsible for most cases of posttransfusion hepatitis is

    (A) Hepatitis B
    (B) Hepatitis C
    (C) Hepatitis D
    (D) Hepatitis E

46. Hepatitis D infection cannot occur without the coexistence of

    (A) Hepatitis B virus infection
    (B) Human immunodeficiency virus infection
    (C) Hepatitis E virus infection
    (D) All of the above

Questions 47–52

The PNP has recently seen Jack, a healthy 12-year-old male, with an uncertain history of varicella-zoster virus (VZV) exposure and no previous VZV immunization. Jack's parents request that their child be immunized against VZV due to the lack of reliable varicella history.

47. Wild varicella virus infection in children is characterized by

    (A) Abrupt onset of high fever with mild systemic symptoms, which subside in 4 days, followed by a pink macular-papular rash of the face and extremities
    (B) Fever, cough, coryza, conjunctivitis, Koplik spots, and coalescent bright red macular-papular rash
    (C) Low-grade fever and mild systemic symptoms followed by crops of red macules that become tiny vesicles, form pustules, and then scab
    (D) Mild systemic symptoms and macular-papular "slapped cheek" rash progressing to a reticular rash of extremities and trunk

Varicella vaccine for universal use in early childhood and in susceptible older children and adolescents is recommended based on the frequency of serious complications and deaths after infection with wild varicella (American Academy of Pediatrics, 1997).

48. Complications of wild varicella virus infection include

    (A) Pneumonia
    (B) Encephalitis
    (C) Secondary bacterial skin infections
    (D) All of the above

49. Bacterial skin infections associated with wild varicella virus are most often secondary to which of the following pathogens?

1. *Moraxella catarrhalis*
2. Group A beta-hemolytic streptococcus (GABHS)
3. Staphylococcus
4. Pneumococcus

    (A) 3 only
    (B) 1 and 3
    (C) 2 and 3
    (D) 3 and 4

50. All of the following are characteristic of varicella EXCEPT

    (A) Single infection usually confers lifelong immunity.
    (B) In general, varicella infection is more severe in children than in adults.
    (C) Incubation period ranges from 10–21 days.
    (D) Lesions appear over a period of 3–5 days.

51. The 1997 recommendation for varicella vaccine administration for this 12-year-old would be

    (A) Administration of two doses of varicella vaccine 4–8 weeks apart
    (B) No immunization at this time
    (C) Administration of one dose of varicella vaccine with revaccination in 10 years
    (D) Administration of one dose of varicella vaccine

52. Which of the following immunizations confers passive immunity?

    (A) Varicella vaccine
    (B) DTaP
    (C) VZIG
    (D) MMR

GENERAL NUTRITION

Questions 53–66

Jessica, a full-term, 4-day-old infant, and her mother, Ms. Shaw, are being seen today on a postpartum visit by the PNP. This gravida 1, para 1 mother had an uneventful prenatal course and uncomplicated vaginal labor and delivery. Both infant and mother were discharged on postpartum day 3. Jessica has been nursing q2h with minimal difficulty and the mother has noted that "my milk is coming in."

53. All of the following are contraindications to breast-feeding EXCEPT

    (A) Breast cancer
    (B) HIV-infected mother
    (C) Maternal varicella infection
    (D) Inverted nipples

54. All of the following statements regarding breast-feeding are true EXCEPT

    (A) Breast size is an indicator of the quantity of milk produced.
    (B) Breast milk is the ideal food for newborns and infants.
    (C) Early assessment and intervention of breast-feeding problems increase the likelihood for success.
    (D) Nurse Practitioners have an important role in the promotion of breast-feeding.

55. Which of the following would be an expected normative weight gain in an infant?

    (A) 1–2 oz per day
    (B) ½–1 oz per day
    (C) 1 lb per week
    (D) None of the above

56. The predominant protein in human milk is:

    (A) Casein
    (B) Lactoferrin
    (C) Alpha-lactalbumin
    (D) Whey

57. The advantages of breast-feeding for the mother include

    (A) Convenience
    (B) Emotional benefits
    (C) Less costly than formula feeding
    (D) All of the above

58. The advantages of breast-feeding for the infant include

    (A) Reduction in frequency of otitis media
    (B) Reduction in frequency of food allergies
    (C) Emotional benefit
    (D) All of the above

59. The two main hormones of lactation are

    1. Somatostatin
    2. Oxytocin
    3. Thyroxine
    4. Prolactin
        (A) 1 and 2
        (B) 2 and 4
        (C) 1 and 4
        (D) 2 and 3

60. Which of the following statements concerning colostrum is *false?*

    (A) It is rich in immunoglobulins.
    (B) It contains maternal leukocytes.
    (C) It begins during late pregnancy and continues for 1 month following birth.
    (D) It acts as a laxative, facilitating the passage of meconium.

61. The use of unmodified cow's milk is contraindicated in the first year of life for which of the following reasons?

    (A) Increased risk of gastrointestinal bleeding
    (B) Increased risk of upper respiratory infections
    (C) Because of its low protein content
    (D) All of the above

Ms. Shaw has concerns that Jessica "is not getting enough to eat." In addition, she says that Jessica's stools were sticky and tarry the first several days and today, "The stools are more frequent, very loose and yellow."

62. Which of the following can help the mother determine the nutritional status of her breast-fed infant?

    1. Home diary of daily weight to determine gain
    2. Home diary of the number of feedings per day

    3. Home diary of the number of wet diapers per day
    4. Home diary of the number of bowel movements per day
        (A) 1 only
        (B) 3 and 4
        (C) 2, 3, and 4
        (D) All of the above

63. Typical stools of breast-fed infants are

    (A) Very loose, yellow, and seedy and occur 2–4 times per day
    (B) Tan, pasty and occur once per day
    (C) Firm, brown and most frequently occur every other day
    (D) Watery, green-yellow and occur six or more times per day

64. Assessment of the breast-feeding mother and infant includes all of the following EXCEPT

    (A) Review of breast-feeding techniques
    (B) Promotion of early supplemental feedings
    (C) Identifying potential barriers to breast-feeding
    (D) Identifying sources of breast-feeding support for the mother and family

65. All of the following statements are *true* regarding the difference in composition of cow's milk versus human milk EXCEPT:

    (A) Cow's milk has a lower protein content than human milk.
    (B) The fat in human milk is better digested than the fat in cow's milk.
    (C) Cow's milk has a higher vitamin D content than human milk.
    (D) Cow's milk has an inappropriate nutrient composition that may lead to nutritional deficiencies.

At this visit, Ms. Shaw wants to know if the medications she took home from the hospital will pass into her breast milk.

66. Which of the following medications is *not* contraindicated for breast-feeding?

(A) Metronidazole
(B) Nicotine
(C) Aspirin
(D) Acetaminophen

Questions 67–73

Ms. Peña, mother of 5-month-old Roberto, has noted a change in his eating pattern. Recently he has begun to require extra nursings in addition to the 8–12 breast-feedings a day he was already receiving. His birth weight was 7.1 lb. His weight today is 15.3 lb. His elimination patterns are entirely normal. He has begun to awaken one additional time during the night to breast-feed. Ms. Peña feels that Roberto may be ready for solid foods.

67. The rapid growth and development in infancy requires

   (A) An introduction to solid foods shortly after 1 month of age
   (B) A need for extra calories
   (C) Supplementation with infant formula in breast-fed infants
   (D) None of the above

68. Which of the following is most important to consider when assessing an infant's readiness for solid foods?

   (A) Developmental maturity
   (B) Weight assessment
   (C) Assessment of mealtime behaviors
   (D) All of the above

69. The traditional age guideline for introduction of supplemental foods is

   (A) Between 4 and 6 months of age
   (B) Anytime after 6 months of age
   (C) 12 months of age
   (D) Anytime after 12 months of age

You note at today's visit that Roberto is able to sit with support, will intentionally mouth a toy, and has doubled his birth weight.

70. Which of the following statements would be most appropriate advice regarding Roberto's readiness for solid foods at this time?

   (A) Continue extra breast-feedings to increase milk supply.
   (B) Give him extra breast-feedings and then rapidly introduce solids at age 6 months.
   (C) Do not recommend introducing solid foods at this time.
   (D) Do recommend the orderly introduction of solid foods at this time in addition to breast-feeding.

71. The AAP recommends the following as the child's first solid foods:

   (A) A single-ingredient, pureed vegetable
   (B) A single-ingredient, pureed fruit
   (C) A single-ingredient, iron-fortified rice cereal
   (D) All of the above are recommended

Roberto's older sister, age 3 years, has been "a picky eater" since 18 months of age and takes a children's multivitamin plus mineral supplement. Ms. Peña fears the same will happen to Roberto. She wants to know whether to give him a vitamin supplement. They live in a town with fluoridated water and do not receive fluoride supplementation.

72. Your advice at this time regarding vitamin supplementation for Roberto would be

   1. No supplementation necessary at this time
   2. Will begin introduction of rice cereal in addition to breast-feeding, and will reevaluate at health supervision visits
   3. Would begin vitamin–mineral supplementation at this visit
   4. None of the above
      (A) 1
      (B) 1 and 2
      (C) 2 and 3
      (D) 4

73. Which is the current recommendation for fluoride supplementation for 5-month-old Roberto?

    (A) No supplementation is necessary.
    (B) Begin supplementation at age 6 months.
    (C) Begin supplementation at this visit.
    (D) None of the above.

Questions 74–78

Chris is a 13-month-old male who is here today for a well-child examination. Chris's mother has multiple concerns about his weight and food intake. Nutrition screening today reveals a child who eats three full meals per day in addition to four or five snacks per day. In addition to his meals he takes in approximately 24–32 oz of cow milk–based, iron-enriched formula per 24-hour period. He drinks approximately 4 oz of fruit juice at each of his snack periods. He eats a variety of fruits, vegetables, meats, and grains. He has not had eggs or whole cow's milk to date. He takes no vitamin supplementation, and juice is made with fluoridated water. He has no known allergies to foods. The parent admits "to lots of snacks and fast food as we are a very busy family—we're often in the car." He is an only child.

74. The objective of nutritional screening by the PNP is to

    (A) Identify infants and children who are at nutritional risk and require a more comprehensive nutritional assessment
    (B) Assess the quantity of food eaten in 24 hours by the child
    (C) Assess parental knowledge of nutrition
    (D) All of the above

On standardized growth charts, Chris's weight has steadily increased from the 80th percentile to above the 95th percentile. His length has remained fairly steady between the 30th and 50th percentile. His weight-for-height is over the 95th percentile. He has just started to walk independently within the last 2 weeks. His physical examination and DDST today are entirely normal.

75. All of the following regarding obesity in infants and children are true EXCEPT

    (A) Many obese children become obese adolescents and adults.
    (B) Obesity in children and adolescents appears to have diverse causes.
    (C) The prevalence of obesity in children and adolescents in the United States has slightly decreased.
    (D) Obesity results when energy intakes exceed energy needs for growth, maintenance, and activity.

76. The most appropriate management of Chris's nutritional issues at this time would be which of the following?

    (A) The PNP should assess parents' basic knowledge of nutrition.
    (B) Schedule a follow-up appointment for a complete nutritional assessment for Chris and his family.
    (C) Reinforce basic age-appropriate nutrition teaching with parent.
    (D) All of the above.

The PNP advises Chris's parent to wean him from his formula and begin cow's milk. Chris's uncle raises goats and his parent wonders whether Chris can be started on goat's milk instead.

77. Why is the use of whole cow's milk discouraged during the first year of life?

    (A) Infants do not like the taste.
    (B) It increases an infant's renal solute load.
    (C) It contributes to the incidence of anemia in infants.
    (D) It is nutritionally inadequate.

78. Which of the following statements regarding goat's milk is *true*?

    (A) It is high in iron, folate, and vitamins C and D.
    (B) It is an acceptable alternative to cow's milk formula for infants.
    (C) It has a high solute load relative to cow's milk.
    (D) None of the above.

Answers and Rationales

HISTORY TAKING AND PHYSICAL EXAMINATION

1. **(C)** A variety of communication techniques are useful in eliciting a history from a client. The close-ended or directive question is useful when one wants to investigate specific points in a history, or when specific information is necessary to assess the client in an acute medical situation.

2. **(D)** A patient who has experienced a recent loss in the family may benefit from empathic responses, which may encourage them to express their feelings. Recognizing that this was a painful experience and responding in an understanding and accepting way will be comforting and supportive to the client.

3. **(C)** There are many challenges inherent in interviewing adolescent clients. To build rapport with the adolescent, interview the adolescent without the parent present. Sensitive issues should be addressed in a nonjudgmental manner. To support adolescents and their competencies, recognize their positive attributes.

4. **(D)** The interviewer who becomes too absorbed in detailed note taking can disrupt the process of the visit by being perceived as uninvolved in the conversation. Instead, try to maintain good eye contact with the client during the interview.

5. **(A)** Obtaining personal information from clients during an interview can create resistance, shame, or discomfort. The depersonalized question is most useful when addressing topics of a sensitive nature, such as those about sexuality or substance abuse. As a nonaccusatory introduction to a question, it is less likely to cause anxiety in a client.

6. **(B)** Open-ended or nondirective questions are helpful in allowing a client the opportunity to provide detailed narratives of a concern or issue. A well-chosen open-ended question can set the stage for the remainder of the interview.

7. **(C)** When information is confusing or when additional information is necessary to take an accurate history, clarification becomes an important communication tool. If the client's accuracy is in doubt, clarification may be important to note any inconsistencies in the history.

8. **(D)** A variety of potential barriers exist in achieving effective communication with clients. These include differences in cultural perspectives between client and examiner, frequent interruptions during the interview process, and lack of continuity of care, all of which may affect your ability to establish a relationship with the client.

9. **(C)** The history of an acutely ill child should consist of questions relating to the presenting illness and the events leading to its onset. The chief complaint is a brief statement of the reason why the patient is requesting care; the history of present illness (HPI) relates the details of the present illness; and the review of systems (ROS) is a checklist for pertinent information on familial diseases, infections, or contagious illness, but has less relevance in the history of this child.

10. **(B)** The first few days and weeks of an infant's life are critical in establishing a healthy relationship between infant and parents. Many parents feel distressed, disappointed, and overwhelmed by the responsibilities of parenting. These parents are at high risk for child abuse and neglect. This patient should be encouraged to talk about her feelings, and the provider should offer guidance and reassurance to assist her with this difficult transition.

11. **(A)** A general principle in the physical exam of a young child is to begin with the least invasive portions first—such as the exam of the heart, lungs, and abdomen—and ending with the more invasive procedures last, such as the ears, oropharynx, and genitalia.

12. **(D)** A young child may be fearful of a visit to the health care provider. When carrying out a physical exam, it is important to take into account the developmental level of the child being examined. It may be necessary to be more creative and patient than usual with a young child. Acknowledging that the child may be scared may decrease the child's level of fear and distrust and enable the provider to be more successful at approaching the child.

13. **(B)** A frequent challenge in the pediatric physical exam is that of examining a fearful toddler. To decrease the chance that the child will cry or resist, exams can take place on the parent's lap. The hands-on component of the exam should take place near the end of the exam, since this is more likely to make a younger child cry.

14. **(A)** The prepubescent child is becoming more aware of bodily changes. Therefore, the physical exam should be performed with attention to preserving modesty. Gowns should be provided and only the part of the body being examined should be exposed. Explanations should be given throughout the exam to decrease anxiety.

15. **(D)** Percussion is a useful tool in evaluation organ size and in detecting dull, flat, or hyperresonant areas. Percussion over an area of consolidation may sound dull; over a pleural effusion, flat; over a hyperinflated area, hyper-resonant. When percussion is performed over the liver and spleen, the percussion note should be dull.

16. **(A)** Percussion is a useful tool in the assessment of the chest and abdomen. In percussing the chest, an area of consolidation may sound dull; a pleural effusion, flat; and a hyperinflated area, hyperresonant.

17. **(B)** A bruit is a flow noise that can be heard on auscultation; it may suggest the presence of an arteriovenous (A-V) malformation. The best places to hear bruits are over the vertex, the temple region of the head, and over the eyes.

18. **(B)** Crackles (formerly known as *rales*) are short crackling, nonmusical sounds heard during either inspiration or expiration. These sounds are a respiratory finding, often due to alveolar or bronchiolar disease, which are caused by the collapse of the peripheral airway, leading to a crackle noise as the airway opens and a thin film of fluid bursts out.

19. **(C)** The Romberg test is used to assess cerebellar function in the neurologic exam. It is best performed with the child upright, eyes closed, with the arms extended in front. By depriving the client of visual input, a child with a lesion on the cerebellum may exhibit loss of balance.

20. **(A)** The Rinne test can be used to assess function of the acoustic nerve and cranial nerve VIII (cochlear and vestibular). It can be performed on older children by using a vibrating tuning fork held close to the external ear and then against the mastoid process. The client should appreciate the former position as producing a louder sound.

IMMUNIZATIONS

21. **(D)** The information from this child's history regarding a household contact who is receiving chemotherapy is important in determining the choice of polio vaccine regimen for this

child. An immunosuppressed person in the house requires using a vaccine that will not compromise the contact's health.

22. **(C)** Polio vaccine should be given at 2 and 4 months, at 12–18 months, and at 4–6 years for a total of four doses at or before the child enters school. Clinicians have three options for immunizing children: sequential IPV–OPV, IPV only, or OPV only. The expanded use of IPV is currently recommended to reduce the risk of vaccine-associated paralytic poliomyelitis (VAPP). Immunization with IPV only is recommended for this child as he resides in the same household as an immunosuppressed adult.

23. **(D)** Each of the recommended polio vaccine schedules—ie, OPV only, IPV only, and sequential IPV–OPV—is highly effective in protecting a child against wild-type polioviruses. When considering the choice of polio vaccine regime for a child, the clinician must also evaluate major factors such as vaccine cost, parent/provider choice, risk of VAPP, and number of injections at scheduled visits (American Academy of Pediatrics, 1997).

24. **(B)** Yearly influenza vaccine immunization, administered in the fall, is recommended for children 6 months of age and older with asthma and other chronic pulmonary diseases. The 23-valent pneumococcal vaccine is recommended for children age 2 years and older who have chronic pulmonary diseases such as emphysema or cystic fibrosis but *not* for those with asthma (American Academy of Pediatrics, 1997).

25. **(B)** Yearly influenza vaccination is indicated for those children with sickle cell anemia age 6 months of age or older.

26. **(B)** Pneumococcal vaccine is indicated for HIV-infected children 2 years of age and older as they are at increased risk of invasive pneumococcal infection. Revaccination after 3–5 years is recommended (American Academy of Pediatrics, 1997).

27. **(A)** Clinicians may encounter some children with uncertain immunization histories due to inadequate documentation or poor recollection by the parent or guardian. In general, these children should be considered susceptible and appropriate immunizations should be given (see Table A27). At the first visit, this 6-year-old child would need to receive DTaP, HBV, MMR, and OPV (or IPV) prior to school entrance. In most children age 5 years of age or older, Hib vaccine is not indicated (American Academy of Pediatrics, 1997).

28. **(C)** If all needed vaccines cannot be administered simultaneously, priority should be given to protecting the child against those diseases that pose the greatest immediate risk. In the United States, these diseases for children between ages 7 to 13 are measles, mumps, and rubella (MMR) (American Academy of Pediatrics, 1997).

29. **(B)** Live-virus measles vaccine, when given as a component of MR or MMR, should not be given to women known to be pregnant or who are considering becoming pregnant within 3 months of vaccination.

30. **(B)** Measles is an acute viral illness characterized by fever, cough, coryza, conjunctivitis, an erythematous maculopapular rash, and Koplik spots. Measles is transmitted by direct contact with infectious droplets and the incubation period is generally 8–12 days from exposure to onset of symptoms.

31. **(C)** Rubella is a mild viral illness characterized by generalized lymphadenopathy, erythematous maculopapular rash, and low-grade fever. Rubella is transmitted by direct contact with infectious droplets and the incubation period is generally 14–21 days.

TABLE A27. RECOMMENDED IMMUNIZATION SCHEDULES FOR CHILDREN NOT IMMUNIZED IN THE FIRST YEAR OF LIFE[a]

Recommended Time/Age	Immunization(s)[b,c]	Comments
Younger Than 7 Years		
First visit	DTaP (or DTP), Hib, HBV, MMR, OPV[d]	If indicated, tuberculin testing may be done at same visit. If child is 5 y of age or older, Hib is not indicated in most circumstances.
Interval after first visit		
1 mo (4 wk)	DTaP (or DTP), HBV, Var[e]	The second dose of OPV may be given if accelerated poliomyelitis vaccination is necessary, such as for travelers to areas where polio is endemic.
2 mo	DTaP (or DTP), Hib, OPV[d]	Second dose of Hib is indicated only if the first dose was received when younger than 15 mo.
≥8 mo	DTaP (or DTP), HBV, OPV[d]	OPV and HBV are not given if the third doses were given earlier.
Age 4–6 y (at or before school entry)	DTaP (or DTP), OPV,[d] MMR[f]	DTaP (or DTP) is not necessary if the fourth dose was given after the fourth birthday; OPV is not necessary if the third dose was given after the fourth birthday.
7–12 Years		
First visit	HBV, MMR, Td, OPV[d]	
Interval after first visit		
2 mo (8 wk)	HBV, MMR[f], Var,[e] Td, OPV[d]	OPV also may be given 1 mo after the first visit if accelerated poliomyelitis vaccination is necessary.
8–14 mo	HBV,[g] Td, OPV[d]	OPV is not given if the third dose was given earlier.

[a] Table is not completely consistent with all package inserts. For products used, also consult manufacturer's package insert for instructions on storage, handling, dosage, and administration. Biologics prepared by different manufacturers may vary, and package inserts of the same manufacturer may change from time to time. Therefore, the physician should be aware of the contents of the current package insert.

Vaccine abbreviations: HBV indicates hepatitis B virus vaccine; Var, varicella vaccine; DTP, diphtheria and tetanus toxoids and pertussis vaccine; DTaP, diphtheria and tetanus toxoids and acellular pertussis vaccine; Hib, *Haemophilus influenzae* type b conjugate vaccine; OPV, oral poliovirus vaccine; IPV, inactivated poliovirus vaccine; MMR, live measles-mumps-rubella vaccine; Td, adult tetanus toxoid (full dose) and diphtheria toxoid (reduced dose), for children ≥7 y and adults.

[b] If all needed vaccines cannot be administered simultaneously, priority should be given to protecting the child against those diseases that pose the greatest immediate risk. In the United States, these diseases for children younger than 2 y usually are measles and *Haemophilus influenzae* type b infection; for children older than 7 y, they are measles, mumps, and rubella. Before 13 y of age, immunity against hepatitis B and varicella should be ensured.

[c] DTaP, HBV, Hib, MMR, and Var can be given simultaneously at separate sites if failure of the patient to return for future immunizations is a concern.

[d] IPV is also acceptable. However, for infants and children starting vaccination late (ie, after 6 mo of age), OPV is preferred in order to complete an accelerated schedule with a minimum number of injections.

[e] Varicella vaccine can be administered to susceptible children any time after 12 mo of age. Unvaccinated children who lack a reliable history of chicken pox should be vaccinated before their 13th birthday.

[f] Minimal interval between doses of MMR is 1 month (4 weeks).

[g] HBV may be given earlier in a 0-, 2-, and 4-mo schedule.

Adapted with permission from 1997 Red Book: Report of the Committee on Infectious Disease *(24th ed.). © American Academy of Pediatrics.*

32. **(D)** Mumps is a systemic disease caused by a paramyxovirus and characterized by swelling of the salivary glands. Complications of mumps include meningitis, pancreatitis, and orchitis. The virus is transmitted by direct contact with infectious droplets and the incubation period is generally 16–18 days.

33. **(C)** Active immunization involves administration of all, a portion of, or a modified product of a microorganism to elicit an immunologic response imitating that of the natural infection (American Academy of Pediatrics, 1997). Many viral vaccines contain live-attenuated virus. The vaccines for most bacteria and some

viruses are inactivated preparations. IPV contains inactivated poliovirus. Hepatitis B vaccine contains inactivated vital antigen. DTaP vaccine contains toxoids and inactivated bacterial components. MMR is a live-attenuated viral vaccine.

34. **(B)** The immediate goal of immunization is disease prevention in individuals or groups of individuals; the long-term goal is eradication of disease. To accomplish these goals, clinicians must maintain timely immunization in the care of infants, children, and adults (American Academy of Pediatrics, 1997). In January 1997, the American Academy of Pediatrics

TABLE A34. RECOMMENDED CHILDHOOD IMMUNIZATION SCHEDULE UNITED STATES, JANUARY–DECEMBER 1997

Age ▶ / Vaccine ▼	Birth	1 month	2 months	4 months	6 months	12 months	15 months	18 months	4–6 years	11–12 years	14–16 years
Hepatitis B[2,3]	Hep B-1		Hep B-2		Hep B-3					Hep B[3]	
Diphtheria, tetanus, Pertussis[4]			DTaP or DTP	DTaP or DTP	DTaP or DTP		DTaP or DTP[4]		DTaP or DTP	Td	
H. Influenzae type b[5]			Hib	Hib	Hib[5]	Hib[5]					
Polio[6]			Polio[6]	Polio		Polio[6]			Polio		
Measles, mumps, rubella[7]						MMR			MMR[7] or MMR[7]		
Varicella[8]						Var				Var[8]	

Vaccines[1] are listed under the routinely recommended ages. Bars indicate range of acceptable ages for vaccination. Shaded bars indicate *catch-up vaccination:* at 11-12 years of age, hepatitis B vaccine should be administered to children not previously vaccinated, and Varicella vaccine should be administered to children not previously vaccinated who lack a reliable history of chickenpox. Approved by the Advisory Committee on Immunization Practices (ACIP), the American Academy of Pediatrics (AAP), and the American Academy of Family Physicians (AAFP).

[1] This schedule indicates the recommended age for routine administration of currently licensed childhood vaccines. Some combination vaccines are available and may be used whenever administration of all components of the vaccine is indicated. Providers should consult the manufacturers' package inserts for detailed recommendations.

[2] *Infants born to HBsAg-negative mothers* should receive 2.5 µg of Merck vaccine (Recombivax HB) or 10 µg of SmithKline Beacham (SB) vaccine (Engerix-B). The 2nd dose should be administered ≥ 1 mo after the 1st dose.

Infants born to HBsAg-positive mothers should receive 0.5 mL hepatitis B immune globulin (HBIG) within 12 hrs of birth, and either 5 µg of Merck vaccine (Recombivax HB) or 10 µg of SB vaccine (Engerix-B) at a separate site. The 2nd dose is recommended at 1-2 mos of age and the 3rd dose at 6 mos of age.

Infants born to mothers whose HBsAg status is unknown should receive either 5 µg of Merck vaccine (Recombivax HB) or 10 µg of SB vaccine (Engerix-B) within 12 hrs of birth. The 2nd dose of vaccine is recommended at 1 mo of age and the 3rd dose at 6 mos of age. Blood should be drawn at the time of delivery to determine the mother's HBsAg status; if it is positive, the infant should receive HBIG as soon as possible (no later than 1 wk of age). The dosage and timing of subsequent vaccine doses should be based upon the mother's HBsAg status.

[3] Children and adolescents who have not been vaccinated against hepatitis B in infancy may begin the series during any childhood visit. Those who have not previously received 3 doses of hepatitis B vaccine should initiate or complete the series during the 11-12 year-old visit. The 2nd dose should be administered at least 1 mo after the 1st dose, and the 3rd dose should be administered at least 4 mos after the 1st dose and at least 2 mos after the 2nd dose.

[4] DTaP (diphtheria and tetanus toxoids and acellular pertussis vaccine) is the preferred vaccine for all doses in the vaccination series, including completion of the series in children who have received ≥1 dose of whole-cell DTP vaccine. Whole-cell DTP is an acceptable alternative to DTaP. The 4th dose (DTaP or DTP) may be administered as early as 12 months of age, provided 6 months have elapsed since the 3rd dose, and if the child is considered unlikely to return at 15-18 mos of age. Td (tetanus and diphtheria toxoids, absorbed, for adult use) is recommended at 11-12 years of age if at least 5 years have elapsed since the last dose of DTP, DTaP, or DT. Subsequent routine Td boosters are recommended every 10 years.

[5] Three *H. influenzae* type b (Hib) conjugate vaccines are licensed for infant use. If PRP-OMP (PedvaxHIB [Merck]) is administered at 2 and 4 mos of age, a dose at 6 mos is not required. After completing the primary series, any Hib conjugate vaccine may be used as a booster.

[6] Two poliovirus vaccines are currently licensed in the US: inactivated poliovirus vaccine (IPV) and oral poliovirus vaccine (OPV). The following schedules are all acceptable by the ACIP, the AAP, and the AAFP, and parents and providers may choose among them:

1. IPV at 2 and 4 mos; OPV at 12-18 mos and 4-6 yr
2. IPV at 2, 4, 12-18 mos, and 4-6 yr
3. OPV at 2, 4, 6-18 mos, and 4-6 yr

The ACIP routinely recommends schedule 1. IPV is the only poliovirus vaccine recommended for immunocompromised persons and their household contacts.

[7] The 2nd dose of MMR is routinely recommended at 4-6 yrs of age or at 11-12 yrs of age, but may be administered during any visit, provided at least 1 month has elapsed since receipt of the 1st dose and that both doses are administered at or after 12 months of age.

[8] Susceptible children may receive Varicella vaccine (Var) at any visit after the first birthday, and those who lack a reliable history of chickenpox should be immunized during the 11-12 year-old visit. Children ≥ 13 years of age should receive 2 doses, at least 1 mo apart.

From American Academy of Pediatrics, 1997.

and the Advisory Committee on Immunization Practices (ACIP) of the Centers for Disease Control and Prevention approved a new unified childhood immunization schedule. See Table A34.

35. **(D)** The patient, parent, and/or legal guardian should be informed about the benefits to be derived from vaccines in preventing disease in individuals and in the community, and about the risk of those vaccines (American Academy of Pediatrics, 1997). Clinicians should provide patients, parents, and/or legal guardians with the opportunity to ask questions and to have those questions answered. The National Childhood Vaccine Injury Act of 1986 includes requirements for notifying patients and parents about vaccine risks and benefits, and mandates distribution of Vaccine Information Statements for those vaccines for which compensation from injury is available.

36. **(D)** A temperature of up to 40.5°C (105°F) is not a true contraindication to vaccination administration following such a reaction to a previous dose of DTP/DTaP (National Vaccine Advisory Committee to the United States Public Health Service, 1993).

37. **(B)** The most common reaction to DTP/DTaP vaccination is local pain and swelling at the injection site. Other common reactions include slight-to-moderate fever, crying, drowsiness, anorexia, and vomiting. The frequency of these common systemic and local reactions is significantly less following administration of DTaP (American Academy of Pediatrics, 1997).

38. **(A)** DTaP postimmunization reactions can be classified from mild to severe. Mild reactions, such as this infant's, include local swelling and pain at the injection site and low to moderate fever. The National Childhood Vaccine Injury Act of 1986 requires clinicians to report selected adverse events following immunization to the Vaccine Adverse Event Report System (VAERS).

39. **(B)** *Haemophilus influenzae*, a gram-negative coccobacillus, can cause meningitis, otitis media, sinusitis, epiglottitis, occult bacteremia, cellulitis, and pneumonia as well as numerous other infections in children. Since 1988, when Hib conjugate vaccines were introduced, the incidence of invasive Hib disease has declined by 95% in infants and young children (American Academy of Pediatrics, 1997).

40. **(B)** Newborns whose mothers have tested HBsAg negative prenatally should receive hepatitis B vaccine within 12 hours of birth. Infants born to HBsAg-positive mothers, including newborn infants, should receive hepatitis B vaccine within 12 hours of birth concurrently with hepatitis B immune globulin (HBIG) (American Academy of Pediatrics, 1997).

41. **(B)** The 1997 Childhood Immunization Schedule (ACIP) recommends hepatitis B vaccination for all infants as part of the routine childhood immunization schedule. In addition, the current recommendation is to immunize all children, regardless of risk, with hepatitis B vaccine by age 11–12 years.

42. **(B)** The PNP should administer the HBV vaccine at this visit as mild URI symptoms with low-grade fever are not true contraindications to HBV vaccine administration.

43. **(A)** Hepatitis B virus is one of at least five hepatitis viruses of humans that cause a systemic infection with major pathology of the liver. Chronic HBV infection occurs in 5–10% of adults with acute HBV infection and in as many as 90% of infants infected perinatally. Formerly called *serum hepatitis*, HBV was originally thought to be transmitted only through blood or blood products. It is now understood that the transmission of HBV may be categorized as parenteral, sexual, perinatal, or horizontal (person-to-person). HBV is not transmitted by the fecal–oral route. The incubation period is 2–6 months, with an average of 120 days. As with the previous plasma-derived vaccine, no instances of HIV transmission have been documented in the current recombinant vaccine as a result of vaccine administration (Centers for Disease Control, 1991). Breast-feeding by a HBsAG-positive mother poses no additional risk to the infant of acquiring HBV infection (American Academy of Pediatrics, 1997).

44. **(B)** Hepatitis A virus, formerly called *infectious hepatitis*, is transmitted by the fecal–oral route and oral ingestion (often from shellfish, water, or food contaminated by sewage). Hepatitis A is highly contagious, and populations at risk include children in child-care centers, persons in long-term care facilities, and those of low socioeconomic status (Moyer & Jenson, 1995). The virus has an abrupt onset with an incubation period of 2–7 weeks (4 weeks average). Chronic hepatitis does not occur following HAV infection.

45. **(B)** Hepatitis C infection is spread primarily by parenteral exposure to blood and blood products from HCV-infected persons. This virus is responsible for most cases of post-transfusion hepatitis. Approximately 90% of infected persons retain the virus, and there are

an estimated 100 million carriers worldwide. The incidence of chronic hepatitis from HCV infection may be as high as 65–70% (American Academy of Pediatrics, 1997).

46. **(A)** Hepatitis D infection causes hepatitis but cannot occur without the coexistence of hepatitis B virus. Infection may occur as either co-infection with HBV or superinfection of an HBV carrier. In the United States, the infection is found most frequently in parenteral drug abusers, hemophiliacs, and immigrants from endemic areas.

47. **(C)** Varicella is characterized by a low-grade fever and mild systemic symptoms followed by crops of red macules that become tiny vesicles, form pustules, and then scab.

48. **(D)** The most common complication of varicella is secondary bacterial skin infection, followed by pneumonia as the second most common complication. Encephalitis, although less common, is far more serious, and long-term neurologic complications are not uncommon.

49. **(C)** Impetigo and cellulitis secondary to staphylococci are common extracutaneous complications of varicella. Superinfections secondary to GABHS can be very serious, and those children superinfected may develop such complications as necrotizing fasciitis and/or toxic shock syndrome.

50. **(B)** Varicella can be more severe, and is more likely to lead to complications, in adolescents, adults, and immunocompromised patients.

51. **(D)** In healthy children ages 12 months to 13 years, one dose of varicella vaccine is recommended and may be given at any time during childhood (American Academy of Pediatrics, 1997).

52. **(C)** Susceptible individuals at high risk of developing severe varicella should be given passive immunoprophylaxis with varicella-zoster immune globulin (VZIG) as soon as possible after exposure but within 96 hours (American Academy of Pediatrics, 1997).

GENERAL NUTRITION

53. **(D)** Flat or inverted nipples can make it more difficult for the infant to latch on in the early days of breast-feeding; however, it is not a contraindication to breast-feeding. The initiation of breast shells in the third trimester can help stretch the breast tissue.

54. **(A)** The breast-feeding mother should be informed that breast size is not an indicator of the quantity of breast milk produced.

55. **(B)** No matter how infants are fed, they commonly lose 5–10% of their birth weight immediately after birth. Once weight gain is established, the expected normative weight gain is ½–1 oz per day. Birth weight is regained by week 3 of life. Infants should gain 4–7 oz/week or, in general, 1 lb per month. Normally, birth weight doubles by age 6 months and triples by age 12 months.

56. **(D)** Casein and whey constitute the protein in both human milk and cow's milk. Amounts of whey protein are similar in each. Cow's milk contains 6–7 times as much casein. The casein/whey ratio of human milk is 40:60, whereas the casein/whey ratio of cow's milk is 82:18 (Trahms and Pipes, 1997).

57. **(D)** The economic and emotional benefits of breast-feeding to the infant, mother, and family are significant. These benefits include convenience, emotional benefits to mother and infant, and the fact that breast milk is ample in supply and cost free.

58. **(D)** Human breast milk and colostrum contain antibodies, enzymes, and other factors that are absent in cow's milk. Breast milk provides protection against a variety of infant disorders, such as otitis media, diarrheal illnesses, allergies, respiratory illnesses, and viral/bacterial/fungal infections (Felman, 1997; Trahms and Pipes, 1997).

59. **(B)** The two main hormones of lactation are oxytocin and prolactin. Oxytocin, a posterior pituitary hormone, is responsible for the milk ejection reflex (let-down response). Prolactin, an anterior pituitary hormone, is secreted secondary to nipple stimulation and is responsible for stimulating the breast alveoli to produce milk.

60. **(C)** Colostrum, a calorically excellent, high-protein, high-fat substance, is produced by the breast for the first 2–7 days after delivery and is high in immunoglobulins as well. Colostrum is replaced after the first several days of life by transitional milk. Mature milk replaces transitional milk by the second week of life.

61. **(A)** Unmodified cow's milk is contraindicated in the first year of life because of its high protein content, poor nutrient content, and the increased risk of gastrointestinal bleeding. During the first year of life, infants should receive human milk or a commercially prepared infant formula.

62. **(D)** A home diary can be provided to the mother to reassure her that her infant is receiving adequate nutrition. Reassure the mother that her infant is receiving adequate nutrition if she can hear the infant suck and see it swallow, if the infant is content after feeding, and if she monitors urine and stool output. In addition, most infants breast-feed 8–12 times per 24 hours.

63. **(A)** Following meconium and transitional stools, breast-fed infants typically have two to four very loose, yellow, seedy stools per day.

64. **(B)** Assessment of the breast-feeding mother and infant includes review of breast-feeding techniques, identification of potential barriers to breast-feeding, and identification of sources of breast-feeding support for the mother and family. The chance of successful breast-feeding increases with early assessment of problems and appropriate intervention.

65. **(A)** The use of unmodified cow's milk is contraindicated during the first year of life. Cow's milk contains about 3 times as much protein as human milk, and it is this high protein content that leads to impaired digestibility.

66. **(D)** Antimicrobial agents taken by a lactating mother often can appear in her breast milk. As stated in the 1997 *Red Book*, "Although important exceptions exist, the majority of antimicrobial agents that might be taken by a lactating mother are compatible with breastfeeding" (AAP Red book, 1997, p. 77). Before offering advice or prescribing medications to the lactating mother, the NP should consult the most recent recommendations, such as those from the American Academy of Pediatrics Committee on Drugs.

67. **(B)** The need for extra calories to support rapid growth and development is the primary reason for introducing supplemental foods in infancy.

68. **(D)** An infant's readiness for supplemental foods depends on developmental maturity, growth rate, and evaluation of nutritional needs. Age alone is not a reliable or accurate predictor of an infant's readiness for supplemental foods.

69. **(A)** The introduction of supplemental foods is an important milestone in infant development. In the United States, the traditional age guideline for the introduction of supplemental foods is between 4 and 6 months of age.

70. **(D)** As this infant has doubled his birth weight and also demonstrates the appropriate eating readiness cues, the PNP would recommend the orderly introduction of solid foods at this time in addition to breast-feeding.

71. **(C)** Single-ingredient iron-fortified rice cereal is often recommended as an infant's first solid food choice because it provides extra calories, iron, calcium, and B vitamins at an age when neonatal iron stores begin to deplete. It is also the least allergenic of the cereal grains.

72. **(B)** In healthy, breast-fed, term infants, the addition of iron-fortified cereal after age 6 months is recommended as it provides iron,

calcium, and B vitamins. With the start of iron-fortified rice cereal feedings, an additional vitamin–mineral supplement is not needed at this time.

73. **(A)** Due to the increased incidence of dental fluorosis, the American Academy of Pediatrics Committee on Nutrition and the American Dental Association have revised their recommendations for dietary fluoride supplementation. Currently fluoride supplements are recommended only for children living in communities without community water fluoridation. Correct dosage is based on the natural fluoride concentration of the child's drinking water and the age of the child. If the community water supply's concentration is greater than 0.6 ppm then no child, regardless of age, needs dietary fluoride supplementation. Infants less than 6 months of age do not need dietary fluoride supplements (American Academy of Pediatrics, 1995).

74. **(D)** The objective of nutritional screening by clinicians is to identify those infants and children who are at nutritional risk. A beginning assessment can be initiated by completing a comprehensive dietary history reviewing daily food records, reviewing standard growth charts, and assessing parents' basic nutritional knowledge.

75. **(C)** Obesity in childhood is a proliferating problem in the United States. Data from the NHANES III survey conducted between 1988 and 1991 shows that the prevalence rate for obesity has risen steadily, increasing since 1965 by 54% in children aged 6–11 years and 39% in adolescents (Troiano, Flegal, Kuczmarski, Campbell, & Johnson, 1995).

76. **(D)** A beginning assessment to identify this child as being at risk nutritionally as well as basic age-appropriate nutrition teaching can begin with today's visit. In addition, a follow-up appointment for a more complete nutritional assessment, for both Chris and his family, can be scheduled today.

77. **(C)** Unmodified cow's milk should not be introduced into the diet before age 1 year. Cow's milk has a much higher protein and ash content than human milk and these differences increase an infant's renal solute load, putting stress on the maturing kidneys. In addition, cow's milk curd is difficult to digest and may cause blood loss from the intestinal tract, leading to iron deficiency anemia.

78. **(C)** Goat's milk has a higher solute load relative to cow's milk and may lead to metabolic acidosis, especially in the first months of life (Trahms & Pipes, 1997). Goat's milk is low in vitamins C and D, iron, and folate.

II

Growth and Development

Cases and Questions

HEALTH SUPERVISION OF THE NEWBORN

Questions 79–86

A 6-week-old is brought in by her mother and father for routine well-child care. She was born at 41 weeks, weighing 7 lb 2 oz, to a gravida 1, para 1, 26-year-old woman, by normal spontaneous vaginal delivery after an induction. Her Apgars were 8/9 and her newborn screens were normal. She received her hepatitis B vaccine in the hospital. She is bottle-fed Similac with iron. The physical exam and developmental assessment are within normal limits.

79. At what age do term infants usually regain their birth weight after the initial weight loss?

    (A) 24–48 hours
    (B) 48–72 hours
    (C) 3–5 days
    (D) 7–10 days

80. During the first month of life, the normal infant's average weight gain should be

    (A) ½–1 oz a day
    (B) 1–2 oz a day
    (C) 1–2 oz a week
    (D) 3–4 lb a month

81. An average 2-month-old child should be able to do which of the following?

    (A) Roll from front to back
    (B) Pass a toy from hand to hand
    (C) Bring the hands together in midline
    (D) Lift the head up 45 degrees when prone

82. The anterior fontanel is usually not palpable on physical exam by what age?

    (A) 6 weeks
    (B) 6–12 months
    (C) 9–18 months
    (D) 18–24 months

83. In a normal infant, the grasp reflex is replaced by the voluntary grasp by what age?

    (A) 2 months
    (B) 4 months
    (C) 6 months
    (D) 12 months

84. In counseling parents regarding dental development, which of the following is *true:*

    (A) The first deciduous teeth erupt between 4 and 6 months.
    (B) The first permanent teeth to erupt are the central incisors.
    (C) Most children have two to four deciduous teeth by 1 year of age.
    (D) Most children have two permanent teeth by 1 year of age.

85. Concerning colic and crying in infancy, which of the following statements are *true?*

    (A) Colic begins in the first 3 weeks of life and usually subsides by 3 months.
    (B) A normal 6-week-old cries for about 3 hours/day.
    (C) Colic affects 10–20% of infants < 3 months of age.
    (D) All of the above.

86. Recommendations for the supine rather than prone position for sleeping are based on data that suggests that the prone position is associated with an increase in

    (A) Bronchiolitis
    (B) Torticollis
    (C) Aspiration pneumonia
    (D) Sudden infant death syndrome (SIDS)

HEALTH SUPERVISION OF THE INFANT

Questions 87–93

A 10-month-old child is seen for a health supervision visit. He is breast-fed and receiving solid foods. His mother complains that he still wakes up two times a night to nurse. His mother is a single parent and works during the day while the infant is cared for by his grandmother. His growth percentiles are 50th percentile for height, weight, and head circumference and his physical exam is found to be normal.

87. Which of the following would be the most appropriate management of this child's sleep behavior?

    (A) Advise the mother that co-sleeping will reduce nighttime wakening.
    (B) Advise the mother to substitute bottle-feeding for the nighttime feedings.
    (C) Advise the mother that nighttime feeding should be unnecessary if the infant is nourished well during the day.
    (D) Advise the mother to try a trial of antihistamines to reduce night wakening.

88. At what age do infants triple their birth weight?

    (A) 3 months
    (B) 6 months
    (C) 9 months
    (D) 12 months

89. By 10 months of age most children can

    (A) Build a tower of two blocks
    (B) Grasp a pellet using a pincer grasp
    (C) Stand alone
    (D) Scribble with a crayon

90. A normal finding in the physical exam of this infant would be

    (A) Genu varum
    (B) Tonic neck reflex
    (C) Esotropia
    (D) Pectus excavatum

91. Appropriate screening during this visit should include

    (A) Urinalysis, Hgb, Hct, lead
    (B) B/P, developmental screening, lead
    (C) Hgb, Hct, developmental screening
    (D) Lead, PPD, urinalysis

92. According to Piaget, this infant is in which stage of development?

    (A) Concrete operations
    (B) Preoperational
    (C) Formal operations
    (D) Sensorimotor

93. Concerning single parent households, which of the following statements are *true*?

    (A) They face greater economic and psychosocial concerns than do two-parent families.
    (B) A rise in births to unmarried women is recognized as a major contributing factor.
    (C) Minority children are more likely to live in single parent families.
    (D) All of the above.

HEALTH SUPERVISION OF THE TODDLER

Questions 94–100

A 24-month-old child presents for well-child care. His history is significant for family disequilibrium, which resulted in foster care placement at age 21 months. He is enrolled in Early Intervention (EI). His foster mother is interested in toilet training him and is requesting more information on how to do it.

94. Successful toilet training requires all of the following EXCEPT

    (A) The child is able to signal the need to toilet.
    (B) The child has reached the oedipal stage of development.
    (C) The child can delay voiding for at least 2 hours.
    (D) The child has the ability to follow simple instructions.

95. A 2-year-old can do all of the following EXCEPT

    (A) Walk up stairs
    (B) Put on clothing
    (C) Point to body parts
    (D) Build a tower of eight cubes

96. A normal finding in a physical exam of a 2-year-old would be

    (A) Lumbar lordosis
    (B) Metatarsus adductus
    (C) Nuchal rigidity
    (D) Mouth breathing

97. Concerning foster care for children, which of the following is *not true*?

    (A) Biologic parents are encouraged to visit children regularly.
    (B) A majority of foster children will be adopted by their foster parents.
    (C) A disproportionate number of children in foster care are minorities.
    (D) Many children experience behavioral or emotional stress as a result of their out-of-home placements.

98. A common feature of 2-year-old behavior is

    (A) Negativism
    (B) Stranger anxiety
    (C) Nonparallel play
    (D) None of the above

99. Recommendations for routine preventive health care of a 2-year-old include

    (A) Growth and development, head circumference, metabolic screening
    (B) Growth and development, vision and hearing, head circumference
    (C) Growth and development, B/P, cholesterol, head circumference
    (D) Growth and development, vision and hearing, tuberculosis

100. Which of the following is a danger signal in language development during early childhood?

    (A) A 9-month-old who only babbles
    (B) A 15-month-old with a few recognizable words
    (C) A 3-year-old with unintelligible speech
    (D) All of the above

HEALTH SUPERVISION OF THE PRESCHOOLER

Questions 101–106

A 4-year, 4-month-old child presents for her preschool physical. The family is expecting a new baby in 2 months. The child's history is significant for recurrent otitis media with effusion (OME), with resulting tympanostomy tubes at 3 years of age, and a urinary tract infection at 4 years of age. She is starting kindergarten in the fall and her mother has concerns about her adjustment to a new baby in the family. Additionally, she has been awakening with nightmares over the past 2 months. Her review of systems (ROS) is noncontributory and her physical exam is normal for her age.

101. Among the following options, what is the best response to the family regarding the child's sleep problems?

    (A) "It is abnormal for healthy preschool children to have nightmares."
    (B) "Preschool children more often have night terrors than nightmares."
    (C) "Nightmares are common during the preschool years and during times of stress."
    (D) None of the above.

102. Which of the following skills would be beyond the developmental level of the 4-year-old?

    (A) Copies a circle
    (B) Recites his or her full name
    (C) Rides a tricycle
    (D) Can count 10 objects

103. Which of the following would be a normal blood pressure (B/P) reading in this 4-year-old?

    (A) 60/40
    (B) 75/50
    (C) 90/60
    (D) 110/80

104. This child's visual acuity using the Allen Picture Cards was 20/50 OD. The best course of action would be

    (A) Referral to an ophthalmologist for evaluation
    (B) Retest in 3 months
    (C) Nothing at this time because results are normal for this age
    (D) Retest in 1 year

105. What anticipatory guidance should be given regarding preparation of this child for the birth of a new baby?

    (A) Children may develop psychomotor complaints as a result of the birth of a baby.
    (B) Regressive behavior is a common response to the birth of a baby.
    (C) Children should be allowed to vent their negative feelings about the new baby.
    (D) All of the above.

106. Recommendations regarding preventive pediatric dental care include all the following EXCEPT

    (A) Fluoride supplementation at or shortly after birth
    (B) Weaning bottle-fed infants by 12 months of age
    (C) No fluoride supplementation to exclusively breast-fed infants

    (D) First dental visits between 12 and 18 months of life

HEALTH SUPERVISION OF THE SCHOOL-AGE CHILD

Questions 107–113

Nine-year-old Adam is in for a physical before starting camp. His history is significant for attention deficit/hyperactivity disorder (ADHD). He has been on Ritalin for the past 8 months, and his parent states that he successfully completed fourth grade. His weight percentile is 90th and his height is 40th. His parent states that he has been lying to her on a number of occasions and has been difficult to discipline at home. She has tried spanking, but he seems to keep repeating the same behaviors.

107. Effective discipline requires

    (A) Harsh punishment
    (B) Ignoring or punishing inappropriate behaviors
    (C) Instilling fear
    (D) Using physical force

108. In addressing this child's current growth, his weight and height percentiles indicate that

    (A) He is overweight for his height.
    (B) His height is greater than his weight percentiles.
    (C) He has appropriate height for his weight.
    (D) He is shorter than he should be for his age.

109. An average school-age child watches how many hours of TV per week?

    (A) 25–30
    (B) 10–15
    (C) 15–20
    (D) 20–25

110. The middle school-age child's cognitive ability would be best described as

    (A) Developing feelings of competency
    (B) Seeing only one's own perspective

(C) Using abstract thinking

(D) None of the above

111. With respect to lying and stealing in school-age children, which of the following statements is *true*?

    (A) They are usually associated with deep psychological problems.
    (B) They are highly correlated with later criminal behavior.
    (C) They often represent a transient behavioral problem.
    (D) They should be ignored to allow the child to "grow out of it."

112. Which of the following is a *true* statement regarding tobacco use and children?

    (A) Fewer teenagers use tobacco than alcohol.
    (B) Fifty-one percent of eighth graders have tried cigarettes.
    (C) Eighty percent of smokeless tobacco users tried it before age 15 years.
    (D) All of the above.

113. When taking a history regarding a behavioral problem, it is best to get information from

    (A) The mother and father alone
    (B) The child alone
    (C) Each parent individually
    (D) All of the members of the child's household

HEALTH SUPERVISION OF THE ADOLESCENT

Questions 114–120

A 15-year-old girl presents to the nurse practitioner with a request to be seen for a physical before playing field hockey. She states that she has been in good health and has no concerns. Her history is significant for sexual activity for the past 5 months with two partners. She has been using condoms with all sexual encounters. She lives with her mother and younger brother and works most days after school at a grocery store. She admits to drinking beer on occasion on the weekends with her friends.

114. The acronym used in obtaining a psychosocial review of systems in adolescents is known as

    (A) TEENS
    (B) DDST
    (C) HEADSS
    (D) CAGE

115. Which of the following is the correct sequence of adolescent female development?

    (A) Growth acceleration, breast development, pubic hair, menarche, axillary hair
    (B) Growth acceleration, pubic hair, breast development, axillary hair, menarche
    (C) Breast development, growth acceleration, axillary hair, pubic hair, menarche
    (D) Axillary hair, breast development, pubic hair, menarche, growth acceleration

116. Preventive counseling for this adolescent should include

    (A) Issues of self-esteem
    (B) Issues of body image
    (C) Relationships with peers
    (D) All of the above

117. Adolescent girls are especially prone to developing which of these disorders?

    (A) Iron deficiency anemia
    (B) Hirsuitism
    (C) Hypothyroidism
    (D) Folate deficiency

118. All of these circumstances define an emancipated minor EXCEPT

    (A) Parenthood
    (B) Sexual activity
    (C) Marriage
    (D) Living on one's own

119. When discussing issues concerning confidentiality, the nurse practitioner should tell the adolescent that

    (A) The parents must have access to all information in the health history.
    (B) Parents cannot access information without the adolescent's permission.
    (C) Parents must be present during all encounters.
    (D) It is at the discretion of the provider to decide whether to release information.

120. Adolescent girls who are involved in high-risk sexual behavior should be screened for all of the following FXCEPT

    (A) Hepatitis B
    (B) Chlamydia
    (C) Rheumatoid disease
    (D) Human papilloma virus (HPV)

Questions 121–127

Tim, an 18-year-old-male, presents to the school-based health center for a sports physical before starting the football season. He has asthma and uses inhalers whenever necessary. His history is significant for a meniscus tear at age 16 years with successful arthroscopic surgery. He is planning to attend college next year. He lives in an intact family with his father, stepmother, and two stepsisters.

121. A routine preparticipation evaluation (PPE) should include all of the following EXCEPT

    (A) EKG
    (B) Visual acuity
    (C) Testicular exam
    (D) Abdominal exam

122. Which of the following conditions would exclude an adolescent from participation in high to moderate intensity sports?

    (A) A functional heart murmur
    (B) HIV infection
    (C) Mild to moderate asthma
    (D) An enlarged spleen

123. Tim states that his asthma has been "flaring up" lately in spite of a new regimen of therapeutics for treating his asthma. What is the *most likely* reason for his treatment failure?

    (A) Street drug use
    (B) Growth spurt
    (C) Noncompliance
    (D) None of the above

124. Of the following, which is a *true* statement concerning risk behavior in adolescence?

    (A) The leading cause of mortality in late adolescence is alcohol-related motor vehicle injuries.
    (B) Substance use is correlated with early initiation of sexual behavior.
    (C) Early initiation of alcohol and tobacco use is a predictor of the use of illicit drugs.
    (D) All of the above.

125. A *true* statement concerning adolescent gynecomastia is that it

    (A) Is associated with later development of breast cancer
    (B) Is a common complaint of normal male adolescents
    (C) Is commonly associated with precocious puberty
    (D) Results from high androgen levels during puberty

126. The role of the nurse practitioner concerning adolescents with questions about their sexual orientation is to

    (A) Avoid talking about sexuality with gay youth
    (B) Refer all gay youth for psychological counseling
    (C) Address sexual orientation in a nonjudgmental manner
    (D) Reassure them that their homosexual feelings are probably transient

127. The most common malignancy in young men is

    (A) Testicular cancer
    (B) Lung cancer
    (C) Non-Hodgkin's lymphoma
    (D) Osteosarcoma

Answers and Rationales

79. **(D)** Newborn infants may lose up to 10% of their body weight because of a loss of body water and because of a decreased relative caloric intake. Term infants with normal nutritional intake regain their birth weight in approximately 7–10 days (Hagerman, 1997).

80. **(A)** The neonate requires 130–140 kcal/kg/day. Given normal nutrition, the healthy newborn should regain the birth weight by 2 weeks of age and gain between ½ and 1 oz a day during the first month of life.

81. **(D)** Although the acquisition of gross motor skills varies in its timing, infants at 2 months of age can lift their heads up to a 45 degree angle when prone. Other developmental milestones, such as rolling from front to back, occur at 4–5 months, whereas fine motor manipulations demonstrated by passing a toy from hand to hand or by hands coming together in midline occur at 6 months and 4 months, respectively. See Table A81.

82. **(C)** The anterior fontanel is the junction of the coronal and saggital sutures. By the time it closes—between 9 and 18 months—it is composed of cartilage and bone and is no longer palpable as a soft spot. When the anterior fontanel closes prematurely, it is known as craniosynostosis. Delayed closure may indicate hypothyroidism, rickets, hydrocephalus, or trisomy-18 (Charlton & Phibbs, 1996).

83. **(B)** Newborns are born with many reflex movements that begin during fetal development. The grasp reflex is a newborn reflex that is extinguished by 4 months, when it is replaced by a voluntary grasping action, which involves reflexive grasp of the infant's hand when a finger is placed into the palm (Charlton & Phibbs, 1996). See Table A83.

84. **(A)** The first deciduous teeth begin to erupt between the fourth and sixth month of age and are usually the lower middle incisors. By 2–3 years of age, about 20 teeth should be in place. The first permanent teeth usually erupt at about 6–7 years of age (Nowak, 1993).

85. **(D)** Crying is a normal physiologic response to distress or discomfort and can create enormous concern and anxiety in caregivers of infants. Colic is a self-limited condition that is thought to be multifactorial in its etiology. It is defined as crying which lasts > 3 hours/day, begins in the third week of life, and improves by 3 months (the "Rule of Threes"). The incidence of colic is approximately 10–20% of infants < 3 months of age. According to Brazelton's study of normal crying patterns in infants, a 2-week-old child cries approximately 2 hours/day, while average crying in a 6-week-old is 3 hours/day (Overby, 1996; Parkin, Schwartz, & Manuel, 1993).

86. **(D)** Researchers have identified that sleep position is a risk factor for sudden infant death syndrome (SIDS). Between the years of 1992 and 1995, SIDS deaths have decreased by 30% due to the campaign to place babies on their backs rather than their stomachs as a preferred sleep position (Willinger, Hoffman, & Hartford, 1994).

TABLE A81. DEVELOPMENTAL CHARTS

1–2 months
Activities to be observed:
Holds head erect and lifts head.
Turns from side to back.
Regards faces and follows objects through visual field.
Drops toys.
Becomes alert in response to voice.

Activities related by parent:
Recognizes parents.
Engages in vocalizations.
Smiles spontaneously.

3–5 months
Activities to be observed:
Grasps cube—first ulnar then later thumb opposition.
Reaches for and brings objects to mouth.
Makes "raspberry" sound.
Sits with support.

Activities related by parent:
Laughs.
Anticipates food on sight.
Turns from back to side.

6–8 months
Activities to be observed:
Sits alone for a short period.
Reaches with one hand.
First scoops up a pellet then grasps it using thumb opposition.
Imitates "bye-bye."
Passes object from hand to hand in midline.
Babbles.

Activities related by parent:
Rolls from back to stomach.
Is inhibited by the word *no*.

9–11 months
Activities to be observed:
Stands alone.
Imitates pat-a-cake and peek-a-boo.
Uses thumb and index finger to pick up pellet.

Activities related by parent:
Walks by supporting self on furniture.
Follows one-step verbal commands, eg, "Come here,"
    "Give it to me."

1 year
Activities to be observed:
Walks independently.
Says "mama" and "dada" with meaning.
Can use a neat pincer grasp to pick up a pellet.
Releases cube into cup after demonstration.
Gives toys on request.
Tries to build a tower of 2 cubes.

Activities related by parent:
Points to desired objects.
Says 1 or 2 other words.

18 months
Activities to be observed:
Builds tower of 3–4 cubes.
Throws ball.
Scribbles spontaneously.

Seats self in chair.
Dumps pellet from bottle.

Activities related by parent:
Walks up and down stairs with help.
Says 4–20 words.
Understands a 2-step command.
Carries and hugs doll.
Feeds self.

24 months
Activities to be observed:
Speaks short phrases, 2 words or more.
Kicks ball on request.
Builds tower of 6–7 cubes.
Points to named objects or pictures.
Jumps off floor with both feet.
Stands on either foot alone.
Uses pronouns.

Activities related by parent:
Verbalizes toilet needs.
Pulls on simple garment.
Turns pages of book singly.
Plays with domestic mimicry.

30 months
Activities to be observed:
Walks backward.
Begins to hop on one foot.
Uses prepositions.
Copies a crude circle.
Points to objects described by use.
Refers to self as *I*.
Holds crayon in fist.

Activities related by parent:
Helps put things away.
Carries on a conversation.

3 years
Activities to be observed:
Holds crayon with fingers.
Builds tower of 9–10 cubes.
Imitates 3-cube bridge.
Copies circle.
Gives first and last name.

Activities related by parent:
Rides tricycle using pedals.
Dresses with supervision.

3–4 years
Activities to be observed:
Climbs stairs with alternating feet.
Begins to button and unbutton.
"What do you like to do that's fun?" (Answers using plurals,
    personal pronoun, and verbs.)
Responds to command to place toy *in, on* or *under* table.
Draws a circle when asked to draw a man (girl, boy).
Knows own sex. ("Are you a boy or a girl?")
Gives full name.
Copies a circle already drawn. ("Can you make one like this?")

Activities related by parent:
Feeds self at mealtime.
Takes off shoes and jacket.

(continued)

TABLE A81. (*Continued*)

4–5 years

Activities to be observed:

Runs and turns without losing balance.

May stand on one leg for at least 10 seconds.

Buttons clothes and laces shoes. (Does not tie.)

Counts to 4 by rote.

"Give me 2 sticks." (Able to do so from pile of 4 tongue depressors.)

Draws a man. (Head, 2 appendages, and possibly 2 eyes. No torso yet.)

Knows the days of the week. ("What day comes after Tuesday?")

Gives appropriate answers to: "What must you do if you are sleepy? Hungry? Cold?"

Copies + in imitation.

Activities related by parent:

Self care at toilet. (May need help with wiping.)

Plays outside for at least 30 minutes.

Dresses self except for tying.

5–6 years

Activities to be observed:

Can catch ball.

Skips smoothly.

Copies a + already drawn.

Tells age.

Concept of 10 (eg, counts 10 tongue depressors). May recite to higher number by rote.

Knows right and left hand.

Draws recognizable man with at least 8 details.

Can describe favorite television program in some detail.

Activities related by parent:

Does simple chores at home (eg, taking out garbage, drying silverware).

Goes to school unattended or meets school bus.

Good motor ability but little awareness of dangers.

6–7 years

Activities to be observed:

Copies a △

Defines words by use. ("What is an orange?" "To eat.")

Knows if morning or afternoon.

Draws a man with 12 details.

Reads several one-syllable printed words. (My, dog, see, boy.)

Uses pencil for printing name.

7–8 years

Activities to be observed:

Counts by 2s and 5s.

Ties shoes.

Copies a ◇.

Knows what day of the week it is. (Not date or year.)

Reads paragraph #1 Durrell:

Reading:

Muff is a little yellow kitten. She drinks milk, she sleeps on a chair. She does not like to get wet.

Corresponding arithmetic:

$$\begin{array}{cccc} 7 & 6 & 6 & 8 \\ +4 & +7 & -4 & -3 \\ \hline \end{array}$$

No evidence of sound substitution in speech (eg. *fr* for *thr*).

Adds and subtracts one-digit numbers.

Draws a man with 16 details.

8–9 years

Activities to be observed:

Defines words better than by use. ("What is an orange?" "A fruit.")

Can give an appropriate answer to the following:

"What is the thing for you to do if . . .

—you've broken something that belongs to someone else?"

—a playmate hits you without meaning to do so?"

Reads paragraph #2 Durrell:

Reading:

A little black dog ran away from home. He played with two big dogs. They ran away from him. It began to rain. He went under a tree. He wanted to go home, but he did not know the way. He saw a boy he knew. The boy took him home.

Corresponding arithmetic:

$$\begin{array}{cccc} & 45 & & \\ 67 & 16 & 14 & 84 \\ + 4 & +27 & - 8 & -36 \\ \hline \end{array}$$

Is learning borrowing and carrying processes in addition and subtraction.

9–10 years

Activities to be observed:

Knows the month, day, and year.

Names the months in order. (15 seconds, 1 error.)

Makes a sentence with these 3 words in it: (One or 2. Can use words orally in proper context.)

1. work . . . money . . . men

2. boy . . . river . . . ball

Reads paragraph #3 Durrell:

Reading:

Six boys put up a tent by the side of a river. They took things to eat with them. When the sun went down, they went into the tent to sleep. In the night, a cow came and began to eat grass around the tent. The boys were afraid. They thought it was a bear.

Corresponding arithmetic:

$$\begin{array}{ccc} 5204 & 23 & 837 \\ - 530 & \times 3 & \times 7 \\ \hline \end{array}$$

Should comprehend and answer the question: "What was the cow doing?"

Learning simple multiplication.

10–12 years

Activities to be observed:

Should read and comprehend paragraph #5 Durrell:

Reading:

In 1807, Robert Fulton took the first long trip in a steamboat. He went one hundred and fifty miles up the Hudson River. The boat went five miles an hour. This was faster than a steamboat had ever gone before. Crowds gathered on both banks of the river to see this new kind of boat. They were afraid that its noise and splashing would drive away all the fish.

Corresponding arithmetic:

$$\begin{array}{ccc} 420 & & \\ \times 29 & 9\overline{)72} & 31\overline{)62} \end{array}$$

Answer: "What river was the trip made on?"

Ask to write the sentence: "The fishermen did not like the boat."

Should do multiplication and simple division.

(continued)

TABLE A81. *(Continued)*

12–15 years

Activities to be observed:

Reads paragraph #7 Durrell:

Reading:

Golf originated in Holland as a game played on ice. The game in its present form first appeared in Scotland. It became unusually popular and kings found it so enjoyable that it was known as "the royal game." James IV, however, thought that people neglected their work to indulge in this fascinating sport so that it was forbidden in 1457. James relented when he found how attractive the game was, and it immediately regained its former popularity. Golf spread gradually to other countries, being introduced in America in 1890. It has grown in favor until there is hardly a town that does not boast or a private of public course.

Corresponding arithmetic:

$$536\overline{)4762} \qquad \tfrac{1}{2} \qquad 7\tfrac{1}{8}$$
$$+\tfrac{1}{3} \qquad -\tfrac{3}{4}$$

Reduce fractions to lowest forms.

Ask to write a sentence: "Golf originated in Holland as a game played on ice."

Answers questions:

"Why was golf forbidden by James IV?"

"Why did he change his mind?"

Does long division, adds and subtracts fractions.

Modified from Leavitt, S.R., Goodman, H., & Harvin, D. (1963). *Pediatrics, 31*: 499.

TABLE A83. NEUROLOGIC DEVELOPMENTAL LANDMARKS

	Birth	3 Months	6 Months	9 Months	12–15 Months	24 Months
Motor	Flexor posture, lifts head prone, hands grasped	Sits: head forward, bobbing, lifts head supine, hands open, retains briefly	Rolls both ways, begins to sit alone, supports (erect), bounces	Creeps, pulls up standing, pincer grasp, sits well	Walks with 1 or 2 hands held, stands alone briefly, releases on command	Walks and runs well, walks downstairs, turns pages singly
Special senses	Regards (vision), may follow 45 degrees	Looks at hands, follows 90–180 degrees	Discriminates voices, localizes sounds	Picks up raisin, "bye-bye"	Localizes noises, localizes pain	Towers 6–7 cubes, imitates scribble
Adaptive	Startles to sound, delayed nociceptive response	Smiles socially, vocalizes socially, follows vertically	Holds cube, palmar grasp, retrieves toy, transfers and rakes raisin	Bangs toys together, pat-a-cake	Assists in dressing, attempts spoon feeding, tries 2-cube tower	Asks for toilet, pulls on garments, spoonfeeds well, parallel play
Language	Throaty noises	Coos, chuckles, vocal social response	Babbles (polysyllables), "mmm-mmm"	"Ma-ma, Da-da," one other "word"	Understands simple command, speaks 1–3 words	Speaks in phrases, names 3–5 pictures, pronouns: "I, me, you"
Reflex	Tonic neck, palmar grasp	Disappearing tonic neck, Moro reflex	Begins voluntary stepping	Parachute response		
Automatisms	Moro reflex, sucks, roots, stepping, supporting, traction: head lag	Landau response, traction: no head lag	Neck righting, blinks to threat			

Reprinted with permission from Moe, P.G., & Seay, A.R. (1997). Neurologic and muscular disorders. In W.W. Hay, J.R. Groothuis, A.R. Hayward, & M.J. Levin, eds. Current pediatric diagnosis & treatment (13th ed., p. 632). Stamford, CT: Appleton & Lange.

87. **(C)** Sleep problems are among the most frequent behavior problems presented to health care providers. When feedings are offered during the night, infants will wake expecting to receive them. Additionally, breast-fed infants will wake and cry more often than those who receive formula feedings (Blum & Carey, 1996). If the child receives adequate nourishment during the day, the parent should be advised to discontinue nighttime feedings to encourage better sleep habits. Co-sleeping, a common arrangement in some cultures, has been thought to cause a higher rate of disruptive sleep.

88. **(D)** During early infancy, the energy requirements for this period of rapid growth is 110 kcal/kg/day. After initial weight loss, the infant gains about 30 g/day for the first several months (Hagerman, 1997). By 1 year of age, infants weigh approximately 3 times their birth weight.

89. **(B)** The infant at 10 months has improved motor dexterity manifested by the acquisition of the pincer grasp (thumb opposing finger). The remaining skills listed are all ones that should be attained by older infants.

90. **(A)** Physiologic bow legs (genu varum) are a common finding of infants in the first year of life and usually correct spontaneously with time.

91. **(C)** Screening tests are a tool used for early detection of childhood problems and conditions (Dworkin, 1996). Screening for anemia is recommended for the infant 6–12 months of age because this is the time period when common congenital anemia and iron deficiency anemia may be detected. Lead poisoning, a condition of potentially serious magnitude, should be screened for when children are between the ages of 12 months and 6 years when there is otherwise low risk. In the absence of symptoms and other risk factors, the AAP recommends a urinalysis during the first year of life, during early childhood, during late childhood, and during adolescence. Routine B/P measurement is recommended in all children > 3 years of age. Developmental screening is an important tool in the early identification of physical, developmental, behavioral, or emotional problems in early childhood.

92. **(D)** According to the renowned psychologist Piaget, children from birth to 2 years are in the *sensorimotor stage,* where they develop a sense of object permanence, spatial relationships, and causality. The 2–6-year-old is in the *preoperational stage,* the 6–11-year-old is in the *concrete operational stage,* and the child > 11 years is in the *formal operations stage* (Dixon, 1992).

93. **(D)** The stereotype of the "typical American family" is changing. Among the many changes cited, one has been the increase in the number of children being raised in single-parent households. This rise is attributed, in part, to the increase among women aged 20 or older having children outside of marriage. Teenagers account for less than one third of all unmarried mothers and children of minorities have been found to be more likely to live with one parent. Single-parent households face greater financial and time stresses than do two-parent families (Smoyak, 1997).

94. **(B)** Anticipatory guidance regarding toilet training should be introduced early to prevent unrealistic expectations and to encourage successful training. Successful training requires physiologic and psychologic readiness. Two years of age is an appropriate time to assess the child's readiness to toilet train. At that time, children should be evaluated for their ability to signal a need to urinate or defecate, for their ability to have dry periods of up to 2 hours, and for the cognitive ability necessary for toileting readiness. The oedipal stage of psychosocial development is usually reached by 3 years of age.

95. **(D)** An average 2-year-old can walk up stairs without alternating feet, can put on some articles of clothing, and can point to body parts. Most 2-year-olds can build a tower of six cubes (Frankenburg, 1992).

96. **(A)** Preschool children have abdominal protruberance, which is caused by transient, normal lordosis. Metatarsus adductus is an abnormality in which the forefoot is adducted in relation to the hindfoot. Nuchal rigidity, a condition in which the neck resists flexion, is an important sign of meningeal irritation. Mouth breathing is not a normal sign in a physical exam and may be due to nasal congestion, obstruction, or adenoidal hypertrophy (Gundy, 1997).

97. **(B)** Foster care is intended as a temporary measure for children who cannot remain in the custody of their parents. A disproportionate number of children in foster care come from single-parent families who are below poverty lines and from minority groups. A majority of these children have experienced abuse or neglect before being placed in foster care. As a result of these conditions, many experience emotional disturbance after their placements. The parent–child relationship is extremely important and visiting patterns are often a predictor of whether children will return to their family of origin (Simm, 1991).

98. **(A)** Temper tantrums are a common, age-related behavior in 2–3-year-olds. They are thought to occur as a result of the toddler's progression toward self-reliance and independence. This stage of development is characterized by negativism and defiance. Management should be directed toward providing anticipatory guidance to families, developing strategies to prevent or minimize this behavior, and allowing children to exercise independence in a positive manner (Howard, 1990).

99. **(B)** The Committee on Preventive Pediatric Health Care (AAP, 1995) has recommended services that should be provided throughout well-child visits. The AAP's guidelines for the 2-year-old well-child visit includes height, weight, head circumference, and developmental/behavioral assessment as well as screening for vision and hearing. Blood pressure screening should be initiated at 3 years of age, cholesterol screening if the history and physical exam warrants evaluation, and tuberculosis if the child is found to have risk factors.

100. **(C)** To detect developmental delays early in a child's life, language skills should be assessed as early as infancy. Language delay is a common presenting symptom of some developmental disorders, as well as a sequela of chronic middle ear effusion (Maxson & Yamauchi, 1996). Three-year-olds should have a vocabulary of at least 250 words and be able to form three-word sentences. Their speech should be intelligible to strangers 75% of the time (Capute, Shapiro, & Palmer, 1987).

101. **(C)** Nightmares, or frightening dreams, tend to occur during the toddler years and peak at 3–5 years of age. They occur more commonly during periods of stress. In light of the upcoming birth of the new baby and the start of school, it is likely that these nightmares are occurring as a result of these stressful situations. Anticipatory guidance aimed at helping this child to cope with her anxiety may help to decrease the frequency of the nightmares (Blum & Carey, 1996).

102. **(D)** All of the following developmental skills should be evident in 4-year-old children: able to copy a circle, give their full names, and ride a tricycle. They generally cannot count 10 objects until they reach 5–6 years of age (Hagerman, 1997). See Table A81.

103. **(C)** Routine blood pressure (B/P) screening should be initiated at 3 years of age. Although B/P norms vary with height, weight, and gender, a normal reading of a child aged 1–3 years would be 90/60 (Headley & Lustig, 1997).

104. **(A)** Early diagnosis and treatment of vision problems can have significant impact on the outcome in young children (Wasserman, 1997). Visual acuity should be tested beginning at age 3 years using either the Illiterate (tumbling) E's or the Allen Picture Cards. Preschool children who receive a test result of 20/40 or below, or those who have a two-line discrepancy between the eyes (ie, 20/20 OS and 20/40 OD), should be referred to an ophthalmologist.

105. **(D)** Sibling rivalry is a universal phenomenon, which occurs as the result of feeling jealous and displaced within a family in relation to a sibling. A common time to experience this rivalry is during the introduction of a new sibling into the family. Common behavior in response to this may be regression, psychosomatic complaints, and aggressive patterns. Parents can minimize this behavior by allowing children to vent their feelings, allowing for time alone with the child, and discussing the advantages of being older (Pakula, 1992).

106. **(C)** Preventive oral health should be a part of all primary care visits in pediatrics. Recommendations from the American Academy of Pediatric Dentistry (Nowak, 1993) include fluoride supplementation for fully breast-fed infants and all children 3–13 years of age who are drinking water with low fluoride content, early weaning to prevent nursing caries or bottle caries, and regular dental visits beginning at 12–18 months of age and continuing at 6-month intervals (Abrams & Mueller, 1997).

107. **(B)** Discipline and behavior problems are common topics of discussion in pediatric visits. To develop appropriate interventions, the health care provider needs to determine the nature of the problem, how the parents deal with the child, and if there are any contributing factors. Effective discipline requires increasing a child's appropriate behavior through reinforcement and eliminating inappropriate behavior by ignoring or punishing the child. The discipline needs to be effective, constructive, and not harsh (Wolraich, 1997).

108. **(A)** The measurement of height and weight plotted on standard growth charts is a practical and common method to monitor growth in children. Although change in the rate of growth over time is the most useful index of growth and nutritional problems, ideal body weight is estimated as the 50th percentile weight for the child's age, gender, and height. Therefore, with a height of 40th percentile, and a weight plotted on the 90th percentile, this child is seen to be overweight for his height (Ehrman, 1997).

109. **(D)** Excessive TV watching has been recognized as an important problem in pediatrics. It has been thought to influence attitudes and behavior in children and has been seen to contribute to unhealthy behaviors including poor nutritional practices. The average 6–11-year-old watches approximately 23 hours of TV a week (Strasburger, 1992).

110. **(A)** Middle childhood is characterized by the development of feelings of competency in one's intellectual and physical skills. Erikson describes this stage as *industry vs. inferiority*. Children who manifest behavioral difficulties may have received negative reactions to their behavior, which interferes with their ability to successfully meet this developmental task (Wells & Stein, 1992).

111. **(C)** Lying and stealing are a common transient developmental problem. Prevalence is highest among 5–8-year-old boys. Although it can represent a psychiatric disturbance, the behavior most often occurs as a result of developmental issues and external influences, such as inconsistent discipline and inflexible, demanding environments. Management should include taking a complete history, offering emotional support and strategies to extinguish the behavior, and referring for counseling if necessary (Prazar, 1997). See Table A111.

112. **(D)** The addictive potential of tobacco has been widely addressed throughout the media and the medical community. Most cigarette use begins in junior and high school years, with 51% of eighth graders admitting to trying cigarettes. Chewing tobacco has also gained popularity among children, with 80% of smokeless tobacco users experimenting with it before 15 years of age (Coupey & Schonberg, 1997). Although more teens experiment with alcohol than tobacco, nicotine addiction causes great concern in pediatric health care (Miller & Cocores, 1993).

TABLE A111. ANTICIPATORY GUIDANCE TOPICS[a]

Age	Safety	Nutrition	Development	Health
Birth–2 months	Car seat Sleep on back or side Smoke detector	No solids	Stimulation	No honey Exposure to second-hand smoke Immunizations
4–6 months	Falling	If bottle-fed, iron- fortified formula No bottle in bed	Rolling Sitting	Fever

9–12 months	Poisons locked up
	Choking on small objects
	Hot liquids causing burns
		Finger foods
		Cup
		Spoon
			Crawling, walking, "mama,"
			   "dada," pincer grasp,
			   social games
				Dental hygiene

15–18 months	Hot water <130 °F Sunscreen Drowning: tub, pail, pool Falls	Set mealtimes Self-feeding Bottle weaning	3–6 words Runs, climbs, stoops Indicates wants and needs Discipline	
2–5 years	Traffic safety Gun safety	Healthy snacks Prudent diet	Peer play Television habits	Family models of exercise, diet Handwashing
6–12 years	Helmets for bicycling, skating Seatbelts Swim lessons/water safety	Fat intake	Chores/responsibility Honesty/respect Sex education School	Smoking Drugs
3–18 years	Sports safety	Junk foods/soda pop Weight control	Responsibility at home Independence	Risk behaviors Exercise

[a] Introduction of a topic is recommended at the age listed; however, reinforcement of the topic is appropriate at later ages as well.

113. **(D)** When addressing behavioral issues in an encounter with a family, it is important to view the behavior in the context of the family. This family-focused approach allows one the opportunity to assess how the behavior affects others and how it is perceived by others in the household. Family-focused strategies in managing behavior problems can help to improve communication skills and foster better family relationships (Coleman & Howard, 1995).

114. **(C)** The HEADSS acronym (Home, Education/Employment, peer group Activities, Drugs, Sexuality, and Suicide/depression) is an important tool to use in obtaining a psychosocial history from an adolescent. Questions related to the topics of the HEADSS format facilitate discussion around important issues in adolescence and allow you to screen for high-risk behaviors (Cavanaugh, 1994; Goldenring & Cohen, 1988).

115. **(A)** Although hormonal changes are complex, the pubertal changes in most children are predictable. Growth acceleration in girls occurs first, followed by breast development. Six months later, pubic hair appears. Menarche occurs approximately 2–2.5 years after and is followed by the appearance of axillary hair (Kulin & Muller, 1996).

116. **(D)** The health supervision visit in adolescence should include discussion of preventive health issues. This includes the identification of high-risk behaviors. Many of these high-risk behaviors are associated with low self-esteem and poor body image (Cavanaugh, 1994). During the adolescent years, children's relationships with peers become important milestones to achieve as they minimize their dependence on parents.

117. **(A)** Adolescent girls are especially prone to developing iron deficiency anemia because of certain risk factors that include poor nutrition with low intake of iron, rapid growth, and menstrual blood loss (Cavanaugh, 1994).

118. **(B)** An emancipated minor is an adolescent who can conduct legal affairs as an adult (Massaro & Wadlington, 1997). The circumstances that can emancipate a minor are marriage, parenthood, military service, living on one's own, and supporting oneself. This status

allows the individual to accept or reject medical treatment without a parent's approval (Cavanaugh, 1994). Sexual activity alone does not constitute emancipation.

119. **(B)** It is important to discuss issues of confidentiality with adolescents and their families at the onset of the visit. By doing this, one can foster trust and honesty and encourage adolescents to take more responsibility for their own care. Although there are no rigid rules concerning confidentiality, it is generally accepted that unless adolescents speak of situations that put themselves or others at physical risk, the provider should maintain confidentiality unless given permission otherwise (Goldenring & Cohen, 1988; Jenkins & Saxena, 1995).

120. **(C)** The American Academy of Pediatrics (AAP) Committee on Infectious Diseases recommends that adolescents who are involved in high-risk behavior, such as unprotected sexual intercourse or multiple partners, should be screened for gonorrhea, chlamydia, trichomoniasis, human papilloma virus, hepatitis B infection, and human immunodeficiency virus (AAP, 1997; Jenkins & Saxena, 1995).

121. **(A)** To assure safe sports participation, the preparticipation evaluation (PPE) exam of a patient should include relevant historical information and a physical exam that can be used to identify potential health problems that may be made worse or could increase the risk of injury to the athlete. At minimum, the PPE should include height, weight, blood pressure, visual acuity, cardiovascular exam (pulses and auscultation of the heart), palpation of the abdomen, exam of the testes, and a screening orthopedic exam. An EKG would not be warranted unless the cardiovascular exam or history suggests that further evaluation is necessary (Andrews, 1997).

122. **(D)** There are rare circumstances that would justify outright disqualification from sports participation. However, a physical finding of an acutely enlarged spleen or liver should disqualify an individual from contact sports because of the risk of rupture. A heart murmur, if deemed innocent, would not disqualify participation, nor would mild to moderate asthma. Human immunodeficiency virus (HIV) infection, because of the apparent low risk to others, is not considered a contraindication to sports participation, unless the individual's state of health does not allow it (Andrews, 1997).

123. **(C)** Adolescent development is mired by many psychological changes. The adolescent often feels invulnerable, which accounts for many risk behaviors during this stage of development. As a result of this sense of invulnerability, adolescents may not adhere to the regimens required of them by a chronic illness. It is likely that this adolescent has been noncompliant with his medication, thereby suffering the consequences of poor asthma control. It is important to foster responsibility in an adolescent for his or her own health, and to give adolescents an opportunity to discuss concerns about their illness (Irwin, Shafer, & Ryan, 1996).

124. **(D)** An important component of the adolescent visit is addressing critical preventive health issues. Substance use and abuse constitute an ongoing problem in adolescence and have been correlated with early sexual behavior, whereas the initiation of alcohol and tobacco use are predictors of lifetime substance abuse patterns. Alcohol-related motor vehicle accidents are the leading cause of death in late adolescence (Irwin, Shafer, & Ryan, 1996).

125. **(B)** Gynecomastia is the glandular enlargement of male breast tissue. It occurs in 40% of 10–16-year-old boys and is a frequent complaint of male adolescents. It results from a relative decreased ratio of androgen to estrogen and spontaneously resolves in 90% of males within 3 years. Although it can be associated with some rare conditions, such as testicular, adrenal, or pituitary tumors, or as a side effect of some drugs, such as antidepressants or marijuana, it most commonly is a normal developmental finding in male adolescents (Chaikind & Shafer, 1996).

126. **(C)** Sexual orientation develops early in child-hood. Homosexuality is a sexual orientation toward one's own gender and is thought to have a biologic basis rather than exclusively a behavioral one. Gay youth are often faced with many stigmas in our society, making them at risk for self-destructive behaviors manifesting as depression and poor self-esteem (Perrin, 1996). The goal of caring for gay youth is to promote emotional and social well-being and good physical health. To meet these goals, the practitioner must be sensitive when discussing all issues concerning sexuality.

127. **(A)** A scrotal mass may represent a testicular neoplasm, which is the most common malignancy in young men (Schlossberger, Kogan, & Shafer, 1996). Adolescents may delay seeking care because of embarrassment or anxiety. The testicular self-exam (TSE) is an important screening tool for adolescent males and should be included in all health supervision visits with the adolescent male.

Common Clinical Conditions

Endocrine and Metabolic

CASES AND QUESTIONS

Questions 128–131

An 8-week-old infant presents with her parents for a well-child visit. Mom had received regular prenatal care. The baby was born at 41 weeks and weighed 8 lb 4 oz at birth. She had physiologic jaundice that was untreated and resolved at 5 days of age. Her Apgars were 8/9 and her newborn screening tests were normal. She has received all immunizations appropriate for her age. She is bottle fed Similac with iron. Parents report recent poor feeding and lethargy. On exam, she is noted to have an enlarged posterior fontanel and a poor weight gain since her last visit. The remainder of the exam is noncontributory and her vital signs are stable.

128. Based on the history and physical exam, what is the most likely diagnosis of this infant's disorder?

    (A) Hyperthyroidism
    (B) Congenital hypothyroidism
    (C) Cystic fibrosis
    (D) Congenital toxoplasmosis

129. An early sign of congenital hypothyroidism (CH) in the neonatal period is

    (A) Tachycardia
    (B) Increased thirst
    (C) Tremor
    (D) Persistent jaundice

130. Which of the following laboratory tests is most helpful in the diagnosis of congenital hypothyroidism (CH)?

    (A) Thyroid-stimulating hormone (TSH) and T_4 (thyroxine)
    (B) Thyroid-releasing hormone (TRH)
    (C) Growth hormone (GH)
    (D) T_3 (triiodothyronine) and CBC

131. A characteristic early sign of acquired hypothyroidism in children is

    (A) Lymphadenopathy
    (B) Growth failure
    (C) Cognitive delay
    (D) None of the above

Questions 132–135

A 12-year-old female is brought in for a camp physical with a history of recent deterioration in school performance. History reveals some emotional lability, nervousness, and insomnia. The family denies any recent stress, illness, medication or drug use, or allergies. Physical exam is significant for a firm goiter and modest weight loss.

132. Based on the history and physical exam findings, what is the most likely diagnosis?

    (A) Hypothyroidism
    (B) Lymphoma
    (C) Hyperthyroidism
    (D) Bulimia nervosa

133. Which of the following test results would most likely be found in Graves' disease?

    (A) Elevated T_3 (triiodothyronine) and T_4 (thyroxine)
    (B) Low growth hormone
    (C) Elevated thyroid-stimulating hormone (TSH)
    (D) All of the above

134. A common ophthalmic finding in hyper-thyroidism is:

    (A) Chemosis
    (B) Exophthalmus
    (C) Ptosis
    (D) All of the above

135. Which of the following cardiac findings is *not* commonly associated with Graves' disease?

    (A) Diastolic murmur
    (B) Tachycardia
    (C) Widened pulse pressure
    (D) Audible bruit over the thyroid

Questions 136–139

A 7-year-old girl presents with her mother with a chief complaint of breast development, pubic hair, and body odor. The family history is negative for endocrine disorders. Physical exam reveals stage 2 breast development with stage 2 pubic hair. Her height and weight are above the 95th percentile.

136. Which of the following best describes this child's physical findings?

    (A) Normal variant
    (B) Precocious puberty
    (C) Premature thelarche only
    (D) Premature adrenarche only

137. A *most* significant finding in a health history of a child with early secondary sex character-istics would be

    (A) A history of thyroid disorder
    (B) Vitamin B_6 intake
    (C) Recent immunizations
    (D) Recent exposure to chemical irritants

138. Which of the following is *not* true regarding idiopathic precocious puberty?

    (A) Idiopathic disease is rare in boys.
    (B) 75% of all cases in females are idiopathic.
    (C) The onset of the disease in a boy may be the first sign of a CNS tumor.
    (D) Idiopathic disease has no effect on skele-tal maturation.

139. Appropriate laboratory evaluation of the child with precocious puberty includes

    (A) Thyroid function studies
    (B) Estradiol levels in girls and testosterone levels in boys
    (C) Follicle-stimulating hormone (FSH) and luteinizing hormone (LH)
    (D) All the above

Questions 140–145

A 7-year-old is brought in to the health center for a 3-week history of nighttime bedwetting and lethargy. History reveals a fair appetite, no recent stress, dys-uria, fever, or a history of urinary tract infections. The physical exam is normal and the urine evaluation shows a urine specific gravity of 1.023 with moderate glucose and ketones.

140. Which of the following best describes the onset of insulin-dependent diabetes mellitus (IDDM) in children?

    (A) The onset of symptoms is usually abrupt.
    (B) Classic symptoms are common in infants and young children.
    (C) It is rarely symptomatic in children.
    (D) None of the above.

141. Which of following is a common presenting complaint of IDDM in children?

    (A) Polyphagia and weight gain
    (B) Ketoacidosis
    (C) Arrested growth
    (D) Nighttime polyuria or enuresis

142. The pathophysiology of IDDM includes all of the following EXCEPT

    (A) Pancreatic beta cell destruction
    (B) Increased glycogenolysis
    (C) Decreased glucose utilization
    (D) Increased protein and fat synthesis

143. Which of the following best describes the metabolic changes that occur in children with IDDM?

(A) Management needs during illness should not change.

(B) Insulin requirements may drop with GI infections.

(C) Insulin requirements may decrease as a result of stress.

(D) None of the above.

144. Which of the following statements concerning the management of children with IDDM is true?

(A) During the honeymoon phase, dose requirements may drop below 0.5 units/kg/day.

(B) Regular insulin is long acting in peak and duration.

(C) NPH or lente insulin is rapid acting.

(D) Daily insulin requirements may decrease during adolescence.

145. Recommended measures to avoid diabetic complications include all the following EXCEPT

(A) Controlled snacking

(B) Regular glucose and ketone monitoring

(C) Measuring glycosylated hemoglobin levels every 3 months

(D) Measuring TSH levels every 6 months

Questions 146–151

Tyree is a 2-year-old African-American child with sickle cell disease (SCD). He presents for his physical exam. His immunizations are up to date. He has received regular primary care at your office since birth.

146. Routine care of Tyree at this time includes which of the following immunizations?

(A) Polyvalent pneumococcal vaccine

(B) Diphtheria and tetanus vaccines

(C) Varicella vaccine

(D) Hepatitis B vaccine

147. Recommended treatment of children with sickle cell anemia includes which of the following?

(A) Routine plasma transfusions

(B) Splenectomy by 2 years of age

(C) Oral prophylactic penicillin by 4 months of age

(D) Oral prednisone

148. Which of the following factors can precipitate a sickle cell crisis?

(A) Infection

(B) Dehydration

(C) Psychosocial stress

(D) All of the above

149. Which of the following is the most common serious complication of sickle cell disease in children?

(A) Pneumococcal septicemia

(B) Lead toxicity

(C) Renal colic

(D) Hepatitis B infection

150. Which of the following characterizes the red cell morphology typically seen in sickle cell anemia?

(A) Macrocytic hyperchromic

(B) Normochromic normocytic

(C) Normocytic hyperchromic

(D) None of the above

151. What is a normal baseline hemoglobin level of children with sickle cell disease?

(A) 11–15 g/dL

(B) 4–6 g/dL

(C) 7–10 g/dL

(D) <4 g/dL

Questions 152–157

Nineteen-month-old Ricky is brought in by his dad for a well-child visit. A review of his growth chart reveals previous weight at the 20th percentile and height at the 5th percentile. His current height is just below the 3rd percentile. The family history reveals that dad had delayed growth throughout adolescence. Ricky's parents are of average height with no history of endocrine disorders. The physical exam is significant for Tanner stage I sexual maturity, four erupted teeth, and a small phallus.

152.   The probable diagnosis of this child's condition is

   (A) A chromosomal disorder
   (B) Familial short stature
   (C) A normal variant
   (D) Idiopathic growth hormone deficiency

153.   Acquired growth hormone (GH) deficiency may be the first clinical manifestation of which of the following?

   (A) Intrauterine growth retardation (IGR)
   (B) Craniopharyngioma
   (C) Down syndrome
   (D) Familial short stature

154.   Which of the following are most helpful in the initial evaluation of the child with short stature?

   (A) History, physical exam, growth curve, radiographic bone age
   (B) History, physical exam, growth curve, trial of growth hormone treatment
   (C) History, physical exam, growth curve, MRI of the pituitary
   (D) History, physical exam, growth curve, bone scan

155.   Clinical signs of children with idiopathic growth hormone deficiency include all the following EXCEPT

   (A) Delayed dentition
   (B) Delayed puberty
   (C) Lower than normal intelligence
   (D) Infantile fat distribution

156.   Which of the following is *true* concerning children with tall stature?

   (A) Marfan and Klinefelter's syndromes are associated with tall stature.
   (B) Children with familial tall stature have abnormal bone ages.
   (C) Children with pituitary gigantism have excessive linear growth rates.
   (D) All of the above.

157.   Which of the following statements would be most helpful in counseling a patient and family about short stature?

   (A) "Don't worry. Good things come in small packages."
   (B) "Try not to focus so much on your height. You'll be OK as you are."
   (C) "Boys grow at a slower rate. Just give it more time."
   (D) "Looking different from your friends must be hard. Tell me more about it."

ANSWERS AND RATIONALES

128. **(B)** Congenital hypothyroidism (CH) occurs in 1 in 50 infants in the United States. It may be due to agenesis or other abnormalities of the thyroid gland, genetic disorders of T_4 biosynthesis, or hypopituitarism (Goodman & Greene, 1994). Most infants born with CH are born with few or no symptoms. Although CH should be detected by neonatal screening, if undetected, signs and symptoms may not appear until 6–12 weeks after birth.

129. **(D)** The earliest signs of CH in the newborn are persistent, transient hypothermia; enlarged posterior fontanel; poor feeding; or respiratory distress with feeding. In the absence of treatment, more severe symptoms can occur, including thickened tongue, hoarse cry, constipation, bradycardia, growth failure, and diminished pulse pressure (Fisher, 1994).

130. **(A)** The diagnosis of CH can be made through measurement of serum T_4 and TSH levels. With primary hypothyroidism, serum TSH levels are elevated and T_4 is in the low or low-normal range (Fisher, 1994).

131. **(B)** Children with acquired hypothyroidism manifest growth impairment early. Muscle weakness occurs in 30–40% of children with acquired hypothyroidism who have prolonged, untreated disease (Fisher, 1994).

132. **(C)** The most common cause of hyperthyroidism in children is Graves' disease. It is four times more common in girls than boys and most commonly is diagnosed in adolescents (Sills, 1994). A goiter is found in 90% of children with hyperthyroidism (Gotlin, Kappy, & Slover, 1997).

133. **(A)** In hyperthyroidism, total and free T_3 and T_4 concentrations are elevated. Additionally, a TSH level below normal can confirm the diagnosis (Sills, 1994).

134. **(D)** Common findings in the eyes of children with hyperthyroidism include proptosis, exophthalmus, lid lag, chemosis, and conjunctival injection (Zimmerman & Gan-Gaisano, 1990).

135. **(A)** Common cardiac findings associated with hyperthyroidism include tachycardia, widened pulse pressure, systolic murmur, and a palpable thrill or audible bruit over the thyroid gland (Sills, 1994).

136. **(B)** The onset of secondary sex characteristics before the age of 8 in a girl or the age of 9 years in a boy is termed *precocious* and warrants further evaluation (Kulin & Muller, 1996). Incomplete precocious puberty can occur with either isolated breast development (thelarche) or pubic hair development (adrenarche).

137. **(A)** Untreated hypothyroidism has been seen in association with precocious puberty, probably due to increased gonadotropin secretion as a result of an increase in TSH (Ott & Jackson, 1989). Central nervous system (CNS) lesions have long been known to be associated with precocious puberty, and hypothalamic hamartoma is increasingly diagnosed as a cause (Kulin & Muller, 1996).

138. **(D)** The idiopathic form of precocious puberty is more common among females and rare among males. The onset in a boy may be related to a CNS tumor. Therefore, it is important to perform repeated CAT scans or MRIs to rule out this diagnosis. If precocious puberty is left untreated, early ossification of the epiphyseal growth area will occur and can cause adult short stature (Ott & Jackson, 1989).

139. **(D)** Laboratory evaluation of the child with precocious puberty includes thyroid function tests, estradiol levels in girls and testosterone in boys, gonadotropin-releasing hormone (GnRH), follicle-stimulating hormone (FSH), and luteinizing hormone (LH) (Lee, 1994). Additional diagnostic testing may be necessary if the history or physical findings warrant further investigation.

140. **(A)** The onset of symptoms in children with IDDM is usually abrupt, with symptoms of less than 1 month's duration. Nonspecific signs of illness are more common in children, which can delay diagnosis (Plotnick, 1994).

141. **(D)** Children with IDDM may present with the classic symptoms of polydipsia, polyuria, polyphagia, and weight loss; however, urinary frequency with nighttime polyuria or bedwetting is a frequent presenting symptom. Ketoacidosis occurs in 10–40% of children with IDDM, but is not a frequent presenting complaint (DuPlessis, 1996).

142. **(D)** The pathophysiology of IDDM results from damage to the insulin-producing cells of the pancreatic islets. This results in decreased utilization of glucose with a reduction in the synthesis of glycogen, protein, and fat.

143. **(B)** The goal of management of the sick child with IDDM is directed toward prevention of diabetic ketoacidosis (DKA). Stress, and the effect of counterregulatory hormones, may have a hyperglycemic or lipolytic effect, whereas gastroenteritis with nausea and vomiting may cause a decrease in appetite, with resultant hypoglycemia and decreased insulin requirements. Frequent blood glucose and urine ketone checks, with the necessary insulin adjustments, are recommended during periods of illness (Plotnick, 1994).

144. **(A)** Many children with newly diagnosed IDDM experience a honeymoon phase within 3–4 months of diagnosis. At that time, their insulin requirements may decline. The maintenance dose of the preadolescent is about 0.75–1.0 units/kg/day divided into two injections. Patients will require more regular insulin in the morning because of typical morning hyperglycemia (dawn phenomenon), which is thought to be due to nighttime increases in some counterregulatory hormones. Adolescents may require increased insulin to achieve adequate control (Plotnick, 1994).

145. **(D)** Regular monitoring of blood glucose and urine ketones is a hallmark of management in the child with IDDM. Additionally, glycosylated hemoglobin (HgbA$_{1c}$) monitoring is recommended at 3-month intervals. In addition to consistent meals, the child with IDDM should have regular snacks to prevent insulin reactions. Only children with thyroid enlargement (20% of children with type I diabetes) should have TSH levels measured once to twice a year (Chase & Eisenbarth, 1997).

146. **(A)** The pneumococcal vaccine should be administered to all children with sickle cell disease (SCD) at 2 years of age and again 3 years later. These children run a high risk of developing pneumococcal septicemia or meningitis, as pneumococcal infections are the leading cause of mortality among sickle cell patients (Ogamdi & White, 1993). Aside from all other routine vaccinations, children with sickle cell disease should receive yearly influenza vaccines (Lane, Nuss, & Ambruso, 1997).

147. **(C)** Poor splenic function predisposes the child with SCD to overwhelming infection from *S. pneumoniae* and *H. influenzae*. Therefore, recommendations for management include oral prophylaxis of the child with penicillin V 125 mg bid until 3 years of age and 250 mg bid after 3 years of age (Buchanan, 1995).

148. **(D)** Vaso-occlusive crises of SCD can occur from a variety of factors including fever, acidosis, hypoxia, hypothermia, dehydration, and psychosocial stress. Management of these crises is symptomatic and includes hydration and analgesics (Kinney & Ware, 1988).

149. **(A)** The most common serious complication of children with SCD is overwhelming septicemia and meningitis due to *Streptococcus pneumoniae* and *Haemophilus influenzae* type B (Buchanan, 1995). Other serious complications include acute chest syndrome, stroke, hand and foot syndrome (dactylitis), acute splenic sequestration, and aplastic crises (Lane, Nuss, & Ambruso, 1997).

150. **(B)** Sickle cell disease is characterized by normocytic, normochromic, or macrocytic anemia with characteristic sickle cells and numerous target cells. The mean corpuscular volume (MCV) is elevated due to the presence of young red cells, and an elevated reticulocyte count is also common (Mentzer, 1996).

151. **(C)** Children with homozygous SCD usually have baseline hemoglobin levels between 7 and 10 g/dL. This level may fall to life-threatening levels during an aplastic crisis or at a time of sequestration (Lane, Nuss, & Ambruso, 1997). Hemoglobin levels above 10 are uncommon, but may occur in infants with SCD in the presence of fetal hemoglobin.

152. **(D)** Growth hormone (GH) deficiency is a condition that affects 1 in 4000 children. Two thirds are idiopathic and the remainder are due to organic or familial causes (Gotlin, Kappy, & Slover, 1997). Other manifestations of GH deficiency include preservation of infantile fat distribution, poor musculature, infantile facial appearance, delayed dentition, delayed bone age, and delayed entry into puberty (Rosenfeld, 1996).

153. **(B)** Acquired GH deficiency may occur for a number of reasons including infections, infil-

trative disorders, cranial irradiation, and trauma. Craniopharyngiomas are the most common tumor associated with pituitary or hypothalamic disease (Oski & Johnson, 1997). These patients may present with headache, visual abnormalities, and neurologic symptoms.

154. **(A)** The initial evaluation of the child with short stature should include a careful history including height and growth patterns of the patient, parents, and siblings; a complete physical exam to rule out any organic pathology; and a bone age evaluation. Children with specific abnormalities found in the history and physical exam, or those where no cause is evident, may require further laboratory evaluation such as: CBC; ESR; chemistry panel, including electrolytes, urinalysis with specific gravity, and pH; thyroid hormone levels; BUN; serum creatinine; and stool exam (Gotlin, Kappy, & Slover, 1997).

155. **(C)** Manifestations of GH deficiency include infantile fat distribution, poor musculature, immature facial appearance, delayed dentition, delayed bone age, and delayed puberty. These children, however, have normal intelligence (Rosenfeld, 1996).

156. **(D)** Tall stature is defined by heights > 2 standard deviations above the mean. Most of these children have familial tall stature and grow above the 95th percentile, with normal bone age. Certain syndromes, such as Marfan or Klinefelter's (XXY), may be associated with tall stature. Growth hormone excess, as in pituitary gigantism, can occur as a result of a pituitary growth hormone–producing tumor (Oski & Johnson, 1997).

157. **(D)** Children who present with short stature or delayed sexual maturity may have significant emotional distress related to their stature. It is important to investigate the child's psychologic adjustment and that of the family's functioning related to the delayed growth.

Eye, Ear, Nose, and Throat (EENT)

CASES AND QUESTIONS

Questions 158–164

Perry is a 16-year-old male who presents with a history of a sore throat, headache, and low-grade fever of 38.1°C (100.7°F) for the past 6 days. He reports a loss of appetite and feeling fatigued. He has missed 4 days of school. He has no known allergies or current health problems. He has taken ibuprofen at home with some relief of his headache symptoms. On physical exam he has posterior cervical lymphadenopathy and hepatosplenomegaly with an injected pharynx and tonsillar exudate.

158. What is the most likely diagnosis of this patient's condition?

    (A) Viral pharyngitis caused by coxsackie virus
    (B) Hepatitis C infection
    (C) Pharyngitis caused by group A beta hemolytic streptococcus (GABHS)
    (D) Infectious mononucleosis

159. Which of the following laboratory tests would be most helpful in diagnosing his condition?

    (A) Heterophile antibody test (monospot)
    (B) Throat culture
    (C) Erythrocyte sedimentation rate (ESR)
    (D) Liver function tests (LFTs)

160. Differential diagnosis of exudative pharyngitis includes which of the following?

    (A) Adenovirus
    (B) Infectious mononucleosis

    (C) *Corynebacterium diphtheriae*
    (D) All of the above

161. Which of the following statements is *true* concerning the epidemiology of pharyngitis?

    (A) Pharyngitis is a common finding in children under 3 years of age.
    (B) Approximately 20–40% of children with sore throats and fever have streptococcal infection.
    (C) Streptococcal pharyngitis is usually seen during the summer months.
    (D) None of the above.

162. Common presenting signs and symptoms of group A beta hemolytic streptococcal (GABHS) pharyngitis are:

    (A) Dysphagia, conjunctivitis, fever
    (B) Dysphagia, muffled voice, drooling
    (C) High fever, oral lesions, irritability
    (D) Dysphagia, headache, abdominal pain

163. Early diagnosis and treatment of GABHS can prevent all of the following suppurative complications EXCEPT

    (A) Poststreptococcal glomerulonephritis
    (B) Cervical adenitis
    (C) Cellulitis
    (D) Retropharyngeal abscess

164. All the following medications would be effective in the treatment of GABHS in a child who weighs less than 30 kg EXCEPT

    (A) Penicillin VK 25–50 mg/kg/day divided bid × 10 days

(B) Penicillin G benzathine 600,000 units IM one time

(C) Trimethoprim-sulfamethoxazole 8–12 mg/kg/day divided bid × 10 days

(D) Cefaclor 40 mg/kg/day divided tid × 10 days

Questions 165–170

Ten-year-old Fred presents with runny nose and congestion for the past 9 days. He complains of a mild sore throat and cough, which is worse at night. His history is significant for viral pharyngitis and appendicitis at age 9 years. Physical exam reveals a low-grade fever, inflamed nasal mucosa, and a postnasal, mucopurulent discharge with malodorous breath. The remainder of the exam is noncontributory.

165. Sinusitis is commonly caused by which of the following bacterial pathogens?

(A) Adenovirus
(B) Respiratory syncytial virus (RSV)
(C) *Haemophilus influenzae*
(D) Group A streptococcus

166. All the following predispose to the development of sinus obstruction EXCEPT

(A) Nasal polyps
(B) Swimming and diving
(C) Allergic inflammation
(D) Viral pharyngitis

167. Signs and symptoms of acute sinusitis include

(A) Facial pain, headache, red tympanic membrane
(B) Persistent cold, periorbital swelling, cough
(C) Enlarged cervical lymph nodes, boggy nasal mucosa, congestion
(D) Vomiting, headache, severe facial pain

168. The sinuses commonly implicated in sinusitis in young children are

(A) Maxillary and ethmoid
(B) Ethmoid and frontal

(C) Frontal and sphenoid
(D) Maxillary and sphenoid

169. Which of the following is appropriate to use as treatment for an uncomplicated course of sinusitis?

(A) Normal saline nose drops
(B) Trimethoprim-sulfamethoxazole
(C) Ibuprofen
(D) All of the above

170. Bilateral, clear, serous drainage from the nose, along with chronic nasal obstruction, is most likely due to

(A) Allergic rhinitis
(B) Epistaxis
(C) Cystic fibrosis
(D) Otitis media with effusion (OME)

Questions 171–178

Nine-month-old Ben is brought in to urgent care for a 2-day history of drainage from his right eye with crusting on his lashes. He is afebrile, but has had a history of runny nose and cough with fussiness for the past 4 days. His sibling has had an upper respiratory infection as well. He is up to date with immunizations and his history is significant for otitis media and bronchiolitis at age 7 months. On exam, his right conjunctiva is infected with palpebral and bulbar edema. There is minimal evidence of purulent drainage. He has dried mucopurulent drainage on both nares.

171. The most likely cause of this child's conjunctivitis is

(A) Viral
(B) Bacterial
(C) Chemical
(D) Allergic

172. An association exists between conjunctivitis and otitis media infections due to which known pathogen?

(A) *C. trachomatis*
(B) *B. catarrhalis*
(C) *S. aureus*
(D) *H. influenzae*

173. Characteristics of viral conjunctivitis due to adenoviruses include:

    (A) Red, watery, itchy eyes with conjunctival cobblestoning
    (B) Periauricular adenopathy, pharyngitis, serous drainage from the eye
    (C) Conjunctival injection, mucopurulent discharge, photophobia
    (D) Red, painful eye with lid swelling, scant purulent drainage

174. The treatment of choice for viral conjunctivitis due to herpes simplex is

    (A) Cromolyn sodium (Opticrom)
    (B) Lodoximide (Alomide)
    (C) Systemic erythromycin
    (D) None of the above

175. The most common cause of a red eye in a neonate is

    (A) Chemical irritation
    (B) *Chlamydia trachomatis*
    (C) *Neisseria gonorrhoeae*
    (D) Adenovirus

176. An inflammation of the lid margin with scales and loss of lashes is known as

    (A) Hordeolum
    (B) Blepharitis
    (C) Chalazion
    (D) Dacryocystitis

177. Asymmetry of a red reflex may indicate which of the following disorders?

    (A) Cataract
    (B) Retinoblastoma
    (C) Refractive error
    (D) All of the above

178. Which of the following eye findings requires *immediate* referral to an ophthalmologist?

    (A) Hyphema
    (B) Corneal abrasion
    (C) Subconjunctival hemorrhage
    (D) Dacryostenosis

Questions 179–185

Fourteen-month-old Michele is brought in by her mother with cold symptoms, fussiness, and fever for the past day. Her history is significant for otitis media two times, at 10 and 12 months, and roseola. Physical exam reveals that the right tympanic membrane is bulging and pink. The remainder of the exam is noncontributory.

179. Which of the following would be the *most useful* tool to aid in the diagnosis of this child's problem?

    (A) Needle tympanocentesis
    (B) Acoustic reflectometry
    (C) Audiometry
    (D) Pneumatic otoscopy

180. Which of the following statements is *true* concerning the bacterial pathogens most commonly responsible for otitis media in children?

    (A) *Moraxella catarrhalis* is the most frequent isolate.
    (B) *Staphylococcus aureus* is the most frequent isolate.
    (C) *Streptococcus pneumoniae* is the most frequent isolate.
    (D) Group A streptococcus is the most frequent isolate.

181. All the following are risk factors for acute otitis media in children EXCEPT

    (A) Bottle feeding
    (B) Race
    (C) Female gender
    (D) Passive smoke

182. Two weeks after antimicrobial treatment is initiated, this child returns with asymptomatic effusion. The *best* course of management is to

    (A) Refer to an ENT for possible tonsillectomy and adenoidectomy
    (B) Treat with an antihistamine/decongestant medication

(C) Evaluate the risk factors and repeat the exam in 2 weeks

(D) Place on chemoprophylaxis with sulfisoxazole

183. A significant consequence of otitis media with effusion is:

(A) Pneumococcal meningitis

(B) Conductive hearing loss

(C) Mastoiditis

(D) None of the above

184. The recommendation for prophylaxis against acute otitis media (AOM) or otitis media with effusion (OME) includes

(A) Treatment with sulfisoxazole 50 mg/kg/day

(B) Prophylaxis of children with >3 episodes of AOM in 6 months or >4 in a year

(C) Counsel regarding environmental risk factors

(D) All of the above

185. The initial drug of choice in the treatment of acute otitis media in this child should be

(A) Amoxicillin 40 mg/kg/day in three divided doses

(B) Amoxicillin 250 mg/dose three times a day

(C) Cefaclor 40 mg/kg/day in three divided doses

(D) Amoxicillin-clavulanate 125 mg/dose three times a day

ANSWERS AND RATIONALES

158. **(D)** Infectious mononucleosis is a common diagnosis in the high school and college years. It results from infection with the Epstein–Barr virus (EBV). Common signs and symptoms are sore throat, fever, adenopathy, fatigue, and headache. Palpable hepatosplenomegaly is a frequent occurrence and palatine petechiae with tonsillar exudate are a common finding on physical exam (Ruppert, 1996).

159. **(A)** The laboratory test used to diagnose infectious mononucleosis (mono) in individuals is the monospot (agglutination slide) that tests for heterophile antibodies. These nonspecific antibodies may not be detectable until the second week of illness. A positive monospot, along with the classic symptoms, usually confirms the diagnosis of infectious mono (Levin & Romero, 1997). A complete blood count (CBC) with >50% lymphocytosis and >10% atypical lymphocytes is also notable in infectious mono (Ruppert, 1996).

160. **(D)** Pharyngitis caused by adenovirus, group A beta hemolytic streptococcus (GABHS), infectious mono, and diphtheria are all characterized by exudative pharyngotonsillitis. Although diphtheria is an uncommon cause of exudative pharyngitis, it should be considered in all nonimmunized children. Exudative tonsillitis may be a rare finding of pharyngeal gonorrhea, but should be considered in all children with sexual contacts (Ogle, 1997; Ruppert, 1996). (See Table A160.)

161. **(B)** Approximately 5% of all ambulatory visits are for pharyngitis. Group A beta hemolytic streptococcus (GABHS) is most prevalent in the school-age population. It accounts for 20–40% of pharyngitis in children and tends to occur in the fall and winter months (Ruppert, 1996).

TABLE A160. DIFFERENTIAL DIAGNOSIS OF THE THREE MOST COMMONLY SEEN CAUSES OF PEDIATRIC PHARYNGITIS

Condition	History	Fever	Exudate	Lymphadenopathy	Other Findings	Diagnostic Studies
Group A beta-hemolytic streptococcal	Rapid onset Few systemic symptoms Seasonal Infection in family	≥100°	Yellow Marked erythema	Anterior cervical	Scarlatiniform rash Tachycardia	+ Rapid strep test + Throat culture
Viral	Rapid onset Systemic symptoms	≥100°	Less likely Swollen, pale pharynx		Cough Congestion Rhinitis Malaise Conjunctivitis	– Rapid strep test – Throat culture
Infectious mononucleosis	Gradual onset Fatigue and malaise	≥102°	White or gray-green Palatine petechiae	Posterior cervical	Hepatosplenomegaly Headache	+ Monospot Lymphocytosis

From Nurse Practitioner, *April 1996, p. 41. By permission of Springhouse Corp.*

162. **(D)** Typical signs and symptoms of children with GABHS are erythema with tonsillar exudate; palatal petechiae; tender, enlarged anterior cervical lymph nodes; dysphagia; headache; fever; vomiting; malaise; and abdominal pain (Ruppert, 1996; Ogle, 1997). Children with fever, conjunctivitis, and exudative tonsillitis may have adenovirus, while those with high fever, irritability, and oral lesions along with vesicular and papulovesicular lesions on the hands and feet may have an enterovirus caused by coxsackie virus A 16 (hand–foot–mouth disease). Findings of dysphagia, drooling, and muffled voice with toxicity may be indicative of epiglottitis or retropharyngeal or peritonsillar abscess, which demands immediate referral (Hazinski, 1996).

163. **(A)** Failure to treat GABHS infection can result in suppurative complications such as retropharyngeal abscess, cervical adenitis, otitis media, cellulitis, and septicemia (Ogle, 1997). Rheumatic fever and poststreptococcal glomerulonephritis are *nonsuppurative* complications of GABHS.

164. **(C)** Effective treatment for a confirmed case of GABHS infection in a child who weighs <30 kg is penicillin VK 25–50 mg/kg/day divided bid × 10 days or penicillin G benzathine 600,000 units IM if noncompliance is suspected. Oral cephalosporins, such as cephalexin or cefaclor, are acceptable alternatives in patients who are penicillin-allergic; however, 20% of penicillin-allergic persons are also allergic to cephalosporins. Therefore, cephalosporins should not be used in individuals who have immediate (anaphylactic-type) sensitivity (American Academy of Pediatrics, 1995; Ruppert, 1996). Sulfonamides and trimethoprim-sulfamethoxazole are not effective against infections caused by group A streptococcus.

165. **(C)** The bacterial pathogens that most commonly cause sinusitis in children are similar to those that cause otitis media. They are *Haemophilus influenzae, Streptococcus pneumoniae,* and *Moraxella catarrhalis.* Group A streptococcus and group C streptococcus are less frequently recovered bacteria. Respiratory syncytial virus (RSV) and adenovirus are *virus* isolates and occur in 10% of patients with sinusitis (Wald, 1993).

166. **(D)** Many conditions predispose to sinus ostial obstruction. The most frequently seen are viral upper respiratory infection and allergic inflammation, although others include nasal polyps, foreign bodies, swimming and diving (Wald, 1993). Viral pharyngitis is not a predisposing factor to the development of sinus obstruction.

167. **(B)** Two common presentations of acute sinusitis in children include persistent respiratory symptoms beyond 10 days or a more severe cold with purulent nasal drainage. Complaints of mild sore throat, malodorous breath, cough, and painless morning swelling of the eyes are common. Headache and facial pain are rare in young children, and severe symptoms may indicate a serious complication, such as an abscess or cellulitis. Boggy nasal mucosae are seen in allergic rhinitis, which is a predisposing factor to chronic sinusitis (Pearlman, Greos, & Vitanza, 1997). Enlarged cervical nodes are not a common feature of sinusitis.

168. **(A)** The maxillary and ethmoid sinuses are most frequently implicated in acute sinusitis in children due to an upper respiratory infection or allergic rhinitis. The frontal sinus is not completely developed until adolescence, and involvement of the sphenoid sinus is uncommon (Berman & Chan, 1997; Wald, 1993).

169. **(D)** Amoxicillin 40 mg/kg/day in three divided doses is a recommended treatment of sinusitis in children. In patients who are penicillin-allergic, or in circumstances where beta-lactamase–positive pathogens are common, trimethoprim-sulfamethoxazole, erythromycin plus sulfamethoxazole, amoxicillin-clavulanate, third-generation cephalosporins, or clarithromycin can be used (Berman & Chan, 1997). In conjunction with antibiotics, patients may benefit from pain relief with acetaminophen or ibuprofen and saline nose drops.

170. **(A)** Allergic rhinitis may be seasonal, perennial, or episodic and is manifested by nasal congestion with seromucoid secretions, postnasal drip, and loose cough. Seasonal rhinitis is also associated with itching of the nose and eyes, tearing, and conjunctival injection. Owing to the mucosal swelling associated with allergic rhinitis, sinusitis may accompany this disorder (Pearlman, Greos, & Vitanza, 1997).

171. **(B)** Bacterial conjunctivitis is a common eye finding in young children. Characteristics of bacterial conjunctivitis are conjunctival injection, purulent drainage, and edema of the palpebral and bulbar conjunctiva. There are often complaints of photophobia and morning crusting of the exudate on the eyelids with difficulty opening the eyes upon waking (Wagner, 1997).

172. **(D)** There exists a frequent association between conjunctivitis and otitis media due to the pathogen *H. influenzae* (Bodor, Marchant, Shurin, & Barenkamp, 1985). This is thought to be owing to the communication between the conjunctival sac and the middle ear with the nasopharynx. The child with mild conjunctivitis, otitis, fever, and mucopurulent rhinorrhea may have the otitis–conjunctivitis syndrome due to *H. influenzae* or *S. pneumoniae*. Systemic therapy alone is thought to be sufficient in eradicating this infection (Wagner, 1997).

173. **(B)** Viral conjunctivitis is frequently confused with bacterial conjunctivitis. It is a rare occurrence in isolated neonatal conjunctivitis and occurs most often in the school-age population (Gigliotti, 1995). Viral conjunctivitis is characterized by redness, itching, and serous drainage and is most often caused by adenovirus types 3, 8, and 19. The triad of pharyngitis, conjunctivitis, and fever may characterize this adenoviral infection (Wagner, 1997; Gigliotti, 1995). A hallmark of allergic conjunctivitis is ocular itching, often accompanied by a history of atopic disease, whereas a red, painful eye with lid swelling and scant drainage may indicate periorbital cellulitis, a serious infection of the structures around the eye (Eisenbaum, 1997).

174. **(D)** Herpes simplex conjunctivitis is a serious eye problem and a rare cause of neonatal conjunctivitis. Herpes simplex virus (HSV) type II can cause corneal opacification and loss of vision. This infection is often precipitated by severe pain, a dendritic corneal ulcer, and herpetic vesicles around the lid and lid margin (Wagner, 1997). If HSV conjunctivitis is suspected, it is important to avoid topical corticosteroid–antibiotic medications because of their potential for serious complications. It is prudent to refer patients to an ophthalmologist for treatment if HSV infection is suspected.

175. **(A)** The most common causes of red eye in order of frequency are chemical conjunctivitis, which usually occurs in the first day of life; chlamydial conjunctivitis, which can occur between 5 days and 1 month of life; and, less commonly, gonococcal conjunctivitis, which may appear 2–5 days after birth (Wagner, 1997; Gigliotti, 1995; Eisenbaum, 1997).

176. **(B)** Blepharitis is an inflammation of the lid and lid margin that causes crusty debris at the base of the lashes with erythema. The two most common causes are staphylococcal infection or seborrheic dermatitis. Treatment consists of daily warm soaks and baby-shampoo-and-water scrubs of the lid and lid margin. An antistaphylococcal antibiotic medication may be applied after cleaning, such as erythromycin or bacitracin (Eisenbaum, 1997).

177. **(D)** An important screening tool in infancy is evaluation of the red reflex accomplished by ophthalmoscopy. If the red reflex appears asymmetric, it may indicate a refractive error difference, a retinoblastoma, or a cataract and warrants immediate attention (Wagner, 1997; Rosenberg & Thilo, 1997).

178. **(A)** Hyphema, a condition in which there is blood in the anterior chamber of the eye, is most often caused by trauma. It requires immediate referral. Corneal abrasions and corneal foreign bodies are conditions characterized by intense pain, tearing, and photophobia. Office exam of the cornea is typically performed with

topical fluorescein sodium and a Wood's light. Conjunctival lacerations, which result in sub-conjunctival hemorrhage, are common and can occur as a result of forceful vomiting or coughing. They commonly reepithelialize without treatment (Klein & Sears, 1992). Dacryostenosis is a disorder of infancy in which a membranous fold obstructs the nasolacrimal duct. The condition appears at 3–12 weeks of age and causes persistent tearing. Treatment is usually delayed until 1 year of age if not resolved (Wagner, 1997).

179. **(D)** In addition to a careful history and physical exam, the middle ear should be evaluated with pneumatic otoscopy to determine the mobility of the tympanic membrane (TM). When positive pressure is applied, the TM moves inward and when the bulb is released, the TM moves outward. If fluid or pus is present behind the TM, the mobility will be diminished or absent (Maxson & Yamauchi, 1996).

180. **(C)** The most frequent bacterial pathogens that cause otitis media are *Streptococcus pneumoniae* followed by nontypable *Haemophilus influenzae*. *Moraxella catarrhalis* and group A streptococcus are less frequent pathogens, and *Staphylococcus aureus* is rarely a cause of acute otitis media (Hanson, 1996).

181. **(C)** Risk factors identified as predisposing children to developing middle ear infections include: being of Native American and Native Alaskan heritage; having craniofacial abnormalities, immune deficiencies, or Down syndrome; passive smoke; and bottle feeding. Males have a higher incidence of middle ear infection than do females (Maxson & Yamauchi, 1996).

182. **(C)** Otitis media with effusion (OME) may be identified following an acute episode of otitis media (OM), or it may be an incidental finding. Although most cases resolve spontaneously, recommendations for OME include continued observation at 2–4-week intervals to evaluate for persistent effusion. When effusion persists, the patient should be evaluated for hearing loss and the need for antimicrobial prophylaxis and tympanostomy tubes (American Academy of Pediatrics, 1994).

183. **(B)** Otitis media with effusion (OME) and serous otitis media (SOM) are conditions in which persistent fluid remains in the middle ear cavity and the patient has no signs or symptoms of infection. It is often a sequela of acute otitis media (AOM). Otitis media with effusion is associated with mild to moderate hearing loss and can be responsible for impaired speech and language development in children (American Academy of Pediatrics, 1994). Studies have demonstrated that about 70% of patients will have persistent effusion at 2 weeks after onset of the disease, 40% at 4 weeks, and 10% at 3 months. Hearing loss may be the only sign that a young patient has persistent effusion (Maxson & Yamauchi, 1996).

184. **(D)** Recommendations for the use of prophylaxis in children with recurrent infections includes antimicrobial prophylaxis with sulfisoxazole (Gantrisin) or amoxicillin in children who have had >3 episodes of OME in 6 months or >4 in a year. Prophylaxis is often given during the winter and spring seasons when upper respiratory infections peak in occurrence (Maxson & Yamauchi, 1996). Additionally, all families should be counseled for decreasing any known risk factors.

185. **(A)** The management of acute otitis media (AOM) involves antipyretics–analgesics and a

TABLE A185. ANTIBIOTIC THERAPY IN THE TREATMENT OF ACUTE OTITIS MEDIA

Drug	Dose
First-line	
Amoxicillin	40 mg/kg/dose divided tid
Bactrim[a]	8 mg/kg TMP and 40 mg/kg SMZ divided bid
Pediazole	150 mg/kg/day divided qid
Second-line	
Ceclor (moderate potency)	40 mg/kg/day divided tid
Augmentin (high potency)	40 mg/kg/day divided tid
Suprax (high potency)	8 mg/kg/day one time
Ceftin (high potency)	30–40 mg/kg/day divided bid

[a]Bactrim is contraindicated in infants < 2 months of age.

10-day course of antibiotics (Hanson, 1996). The first line treatment of AOM includes amoxicillin 40 mg/kg/day in three divided doses. The dose of medication is determined by the *weight* of the child. Amoxicillin is relatively inexpensive and effective against the majority of pathogens. Other agents such as amoxicillin-clavulanate (Augmentin), trimethoprim-sulfamethoxazole (Bactrim), or erythromycin-sulfisoxazole (Pedi-azole) may be considered in patients who have taken amoxicillin recently. In areas where there is a high incidence of beta-lactamase–resistant organisms, an alternative antimicrobial should be considered (Maxson & Yamauchi, 1996).

Hematologic and Immunologic

Questions 186–192

Ariel, a 6-month-old, is brought into a walk-in clinic with a 2-day history of fever and irritability. Her parents state she has had no other symptoms except for a poor appetite and she has received no medications except for a dose of Tylenol. On exam, she is fussy but consolable by her parents. Her vital signs are normal with the exception of a rectal temperature of 39.7°C (103.4°F). The physical exam is normal and no source for the fever is evident.

186. Which of the following factors increases a child's risk of developing bacteremia?

    (A) A white blood count (WBC) > 15,000/mL
    (B) Young age
    (C) A fever > 39.0°C (102.2°F)
    (D) All of the above

187. The organism most frequently responsible for occult bacteremia in children 3–36 months of age is

    (A) *Salmonella*
    (B) *Haemophilus influenzae*
    (C) *Streptococcus pneumoniae*
    (D) *Escherichia coli*

188. To reduce fever in this 6-month-old, the appropriate antipyretic measures would be

    (A) Sponging with cool water
    (B) 10–15 mg/kg acetaminophen
    (C) 20 mg/kg acetylsalicylic acid
    (D) 50 mg/kg ibuprofen

189. The leading cause of fever of undetermined origin (FUO) in children is

    (A) Infection
    (B) Neoplasm
    (C) Autoimmune disease
    (D) Connective tissue disease

190. Fever is defined by which of the following temperature readings?

    (A) Infrared temperature of 37.2°C (99.0°F)
    (B) Oral temperature of 37.8°C (100.0°F)
    (C) Axillary temperature of 37.2°C (99.0°F)
    (D) Rectal temperature of 38.0°C (100.4°F)

191. Which of the following children warrants aggressive antipyretic therapy?

    (A) A 6-year-old with a temperature of 39.4°C (103.0°F) and pharyngitis
    (B) A 13-month-old with a temperature of 38.3°C (101.0°F) and a history of febrile seizures
    (C) A 10-month-old with a temperature of 38.6°C (102.6°F) and otitis
    (D) A 3-year-old with a temperature of 38.8°C (102.0°F) and diarrhea

192. Initial management of this child should include which of the following laboratory tests?

    (A) WBC, blood culture, urinalysis, urine culture
    (B) CBC, stool smear, blood culture, lumbar puncture
    (C) WBC, blood culture, tuberculin skin test, urinalysis
    (D) CBC, ESR, liver enzymes, throat culture

Questions 193–198

Harry is an 8 lb 2 oz Caucasian infant who was delivered at term without complications and is in to be evaluated at 4 days of age. He was discharged with his mother at 42 hours of age and she has been breast-feeding him since delivery. He was initially slow to latch on, but recent nursing has been successful. He has been nursing an average of 10 times a day. His mother noticed he was yellow on day 3. He is voiding well and has had four meconium stools since birth. His physical exam is entirely normal. A total serum bilirubin drawn is 14.8 mg/dL with a direct bilirubin of 1.0 mg/dL.

193.   What factors are known to promote high early serum bilirubin concentrations?

(A) Artificial feeding
(B) Unsupplemented breast-feeding
(C) Hemolysis
(D) Type O blood in a mother

194.   The next step in management of this infant includes

(A) Stopping breast-feeding the infant at this time
(B) Laboratory evaluation of liver function
(C) Referring the infant to the ER for admission
(D) Laboratory evaluation of hematocrit, hemoglobin, and peripheral blood smear

195.   All the following diagnostic studies are helpful in determining hemolytic disease of the newborn EXCEPT

(A) Hemoglobin and hematocrit
(B) Reticulocyte count
(C) Blood smear
(D) ABO typing

196.   The serum bilirubin concentration of this child is considered to be

(A) Above physiologic limits
(B) Within physiologic limits
(C) Prolonged hyperbilirubinemia
(D) Early hyperbilirubinemia

197.   Which of the following is a sign of inadequate breast milk intake in the first few weeks of life?

(A) 12% weight loss from birth weight in the first week of life
(B) Nursing 8–10 times in 24 hours
(C) 6 wet diapers per day
(D) None of the above

198.   Which of the following laboratory data suggests the need for home phototherapy in an infant without hemolysis?

(A) 17 mg/dL at age 2 days
(B) 19 mg/dL at age 3 days
(C) 22 mg/dL at age 4 days
(D) All of the above

Questions 199–204

A 15-year-old female is brought in by her foster parent for evaluation of weight loss, fatigue, and anorexia for the past 3 weeks. Her history is significant for sexual abuse by a stepbrother at age 11, with poor school performance, drug experimentation, and a recent period of homelessness. She has not received any routine health care in the past 5 years. Physical exam reveals generalized lymphadenopathy with hepatosplenomegaly. Based on her history, risk factors and physical exam, she is counseled to receive a serologic test for the antibody to human immunodeficiency virus (HIV) at this time.

199.   Which of the following statements is *not true* regarding the transmission of acquired immunodeficiency syndrome (AIDS) in children?

(A) Mother–infant transmission can occur during breast feeding.
(B) Transmission is vertical in 85–90% of pediatric cases.
(C) Heterosexual contact is a common mode of transmission among adolescents.
(D) 75% of women with HIV transmit it to their offspring.

200. Which of the following immunization modifications is recommended for HIV-seropositive children?

(A) Eliminate all live virus vaccines
(B) Substitute oral polio for inactivated poliovirus vaccine
(C) Substitute Td for DPT
(D) Administer pneumococcal vaccine after age 6 months

201. Which of the following is *not* a common clinical presentation of AIDS in children?

(A) Kaposi's sarcoma
(B) Failure to thrive (FTT)
(C) Recurrent bacterial pneumonia
(D) Recurrent or chronic thrush

202. In addition to antiretroviral therapy, children with HIV should receive which of the following as routine therapy?

(A) Prophylaxis for *Pneumocystis carinii* infection
(B) Tuberculosis prophylaxis
(C) Clotrimazole therapy
(D) Prophylaxis for Kaposi's sarcoma

203. Which of the following precautions should be recommended to the caregivers about HIV transmission?

(A) HIV-positive children should be excluded from day-care settings.
(B) HIV-positive children should be isolated from school when ill with infections.
(C) Universal precautions should be implemented in the care of all children.
(D) All of the above.

204. Current recommendations to reduce the risk of prenatal transmission of HIV infection include

(A) Amphotericin B therapy to all HIV-infected pregnant women
(B) Cesarean section to deliver all HIV-infected pregnant women
(C) Administration of zidovudine (ZDV) to HIV-infected pregnant women

(D) Routine delivery at 36 weeks of all HIV-infected pregnant women

Questions 205–208

A 3-year, 3-month-old Caucasian male is brought in by his aunt for evaluation of leg pain and abdominal pain over the past 6 weeks. At times he refuses to walk. His aunt has noticed that he seems lethargic and has had a diminished appetite. He has had no history of trauma or recent illnesses or immunizations. On exam he appears pale with a temperature of 37.8°C (100.2 F). Range of motion of his knees and strength in his legs are decreased. He has generalized cervical adenopathy.

205. Which of the following sets of laboratory results is abnormal?

(A) Hemoglobin 6.5 g/dL; WBC 2400/mm^3; platelets 50,000; reticulocyte count 0.5%
(B) Hemoglobin 12.0 g/dL; WBC 11,500/mm^3; platelets 160,000; reticulocyte count 1.0%
(C) Hemoglobin 12.0 g/dL; WBC 11,500/mm^3; platelets 25,000; reticulocyte count 1.0%
(D) None of the above

206. Which of the following statements is *not true* concerning leukemia in children?

(A) Acute lymphoblastic leukemia is the most common malignancy in childhood.
(B) The peak age of onset is 4 years of age.
(C) The most common presenting symptom is significant weight loss.
(D) The disease is more common in white than nonwhite children.

207. Patients receiving therapy for acute lymphoblastic leukemia (ALL) should be prophylaxed against

(A) *Candida albicans*
(B) *Clostridium difficile*
(C) Rubeola
(D) *Pneumocystis carinii*

208. Of the following, which is the major cause of morbidity and mortality in the child with leukemia?

(A) Bowel obstruction
(B) Infection
(C) Renal failure
(D) Hemorrhage

Questions 209–213

Eleven-year-old Sasha is brought in for her precamp physical by her mother. The history reveals that she has had intermittent headaches for the past 3 months. She complains of fatigue and declining school performance. Her headaches have been progressively worsening, and morning vomiting has occurred with some headache relief. Her mother denies any recent illness, stress, or exposure to communicable diseases. She has been taking ibuprofen for pain relief.

209. Which of the following statements is *true* concerning brain tumors in children?

(A) Brain tumors are a rare form of cancer in children.
(B) Malignancies are the leading cause of death in children.
(C) Seizures are the most common presenting complaint.
(D) Astrocytoma is the most common pediatric brain tumor.

210. Headache symptoms in this child are most likely due to:

(A) Stress
(B) Migraines
(C) Increased intracranial pressure
(D) Drug toxicity

211. A likely cause of a large abdominal mass in a 2-year-old is

(A) Retinoblastoma
(B) Wilms' tumor
(C) Non-Hodgkin's lymphoma
(D) Adrenal carcinoma

212. A white pupillary reflex (leukocoria) may be indicative of which of the following conditions?

(A) Retinoblastoma
(B) Strabismus
(C) Medulloblastoma
(D) Normal findings

213. Psychosocial issues that are sequelae to the child with cancer include

(A) School failure
(B) Changes in family relationships
(C) Economic burden
(D) All of the above

Questions 214–218

Twenty-month-old Graeme is in for evaluation of crankiness, constipation, and anorexia. He lives with his grandmother, who has tried some herbal remedies at home. He was last seen at 10 months for a physical exam. History reveals that Graeme had been living with his grandmother since he was 8 months old, in an old house which is being renovated by the landlord. Laboratory evaluation of Graeme reveals a blood lead level of 27 µg/dL.

214. Which age group is at the greatest risk of developing lead toxicity?

(A) 3–6 months
(B) 6–12 months
(C) 1–3 years
(D) 3–5 years

215. What is the current Centers for Disease Control (CDC) recommendation concerning the frequency of routine screening for lead poisoning?

(A) Routine screening only of those children who are symptomatic
(B) No routine screening unless risk factors are identified
(C) Routine screening at 12 and 24 months in asymptomatic children with low risk
(D) Routine screening at 6 and 36 months in asymptomatic children with low risk

216. Which of the following whole blood lead levels warrants medical evaluation and consideration of therapy?

(A) 4 µg/dL
(B) 8 µg/dL

(C) 15 µg/dL

(D) 25 µg/dL

217. All the following are potential sources of lead exposure EXCEPT

(A) Rosehips
(B) Colored newsprint
(C) Water
(D) Soil

218. Which of the following findings on a physical exam should lead to consideration of lead screening?

(A) A behavior disorder in a 4-year-old
(B) A hearing loss in a 2.5-year-old
(C) Unexplained seizures in a 6-year-old
(D) All of the above

Questions 219–224

Carlos is a 27-month-old, Hispanic male, who is brought in for a well-child check by his mother. Prenatal history reveals a normal pregnancy and labor, and delivery at 39.5 weeks, with a birth weight of 7 lb 2 oz, and no postnatal complications. Mother and baby were discharged at 40 hours of age. Carlos's mother reports that he has been healthy except for three episodes of URI and two episodes of OM in his first year of life. Carlos is described as a picky eater and the history reveals that he drinks up to 48 ounces of whole milk each day from a bottle and some fruit juice from the cup. He has had normal growth and development and a review of systems is unremarkable. Physical exam reveals an alert, active toddler who is well nourished. His growth parameters are in the 60th and 75th percentiles, respectively, for height and weight. Physical findings are unremarkable except for pallor of his skin and conjunctiva.

219. In the diet history, which of the following *most* needs further evaluation?

(A) Cholesterol intake
(B) Fiber intake

(C) Daily intake of red meats and green leafy vegetables
(D) Daily intake of citrus juice

220. Other questions in the history that would be *most* important to ask concerning his diet include

(A) Family history of anemia
(B) Amounts of fiber in his diet
(C) Use of vitamin supplements
(D) None of the above

221. Which of the following tests is the most appropriate to order at this time?

(A) Coombs' test
(B) Indirect and direct bilirubin
(C) Liver function tests (LFTs)
(D) Hematocrit, hemoglobin, mean corpuscular volume (MCV), and blood smear

222. Physical findings consistent with mild anemia include

(A) Pallor and fatigue
(B) Splenic enlargement
(C) Tachycardia and tachypnea
(D) Bruises, petechiae, and mucosal bleeding

223. What is the best interpretation of the following laboratory test results: Hgb 9.0 g/dL; Hct 28.5%; MCV 70 mm^3; reticulocyte count 0.5% with hypochromic, microcytic red cells?

(A) Folate deficiency
(B) Sickle cell anemia
(C) Iron deficiency anemia
(D) Chronic infection

224. Which of the following is the best treatment for Carlos's disorder?

(A) Dietary restriction of whole milk
(B) A therapeutic trial of elemental iron
(C) An increase of fiber in the diet
(D) One multivitamin a day for 30 days

ANSWERS AND RATIONALES

186. (D) The risk of occult bacteremia in children is increased with a fever > 39.0°C (102.2°F), WBC counts >15,000 or <5,000, and in those who are less than 24 months of age (Wilson, 1995; Baraff et al., 1993).

187. (C) The most common organism implicated in occult bacteremia is *Streptococcus pneumoniae,* which accounts for 70–90% of cases. *Haemophilus influenzae, Salmonella*, and *Neisseria meningitidis* account for the remainder of cases (Oski, 1997; Avner, 1997).

188. (B) Acetaminophen is the drug of choice in reducing fever in children. The recommended dose is 10–15 mg/kg. Although both ibuprofen and salicylic acid are effective at reducing fever, aspirin (acetylsalicylic acid) is associated with Reye's syndrome, interferes with clotting, and is irritating to the stomach. Ibuprofen may cause gastrointestinal upset as well.

189. (A) A fever persisting beyond 5–7 days is known as a fever of unknown origin (FUO). Infection is the leading cause of FUO in all ages, accounting for 50% of cases in children. Common bacterial infections in febrile children include otitis, pneumonia, meningitis, osteomyelitis, gastroenteritis, and urinary tract infections (Wilson, 1995). Connective tissue disorders and malignancies account for the remainder of cases in children.

190. (D) Confusion exists on the lack of a consistent definition of fever. Fever is defined as an oral temperature of 37.7°C (100.0°F), axillary temperature of 37.2°C (99.0°F), and rectal temperature of 38°C (100.4°F). Infrared thermometers aimed at the tympanic membrane are popular; however, the glass thermometer remains the gold standard for the measurement of temperature (Wilson, 1995).

191. (B) Children with a history of febrile seizures, neurologic disorders, metabolic disorders, and cardiac or pulmonary problems warrant aggressive fever management. About 25–30% of children with an initial febrile seizure will have another episode within 6–12 months (Wilson, 1995).

192. (A) Although no single laboratory test can be used to predict serious illness in febrile children, a white blood count (WBC), blood culture, urinalysis, and urine culture are appropriate diagnostic tools in the evaluation of febrile children. Other laboratory tests such as stool culture, lumbar puncture, chest x-ray, and tuberculin skin testing may be necessary in situations where the history and physical findings warrant it (Oski, 1997).

193. (C) A number of factors can promote high early serum bilirubin concentrations. These include hemolysis, hematomas, poor early feeding practices, delayed onset of stooling, Asian race, and maternal diabetes (Oski, 1992; Gartner, 1994). Formula feeding alone is not a risk factor and early, frequent, unsupplemented breast-feeding prevents exaggeration of early physiologic jaundice. Infants of mothers with blood type O have lower frequency of significant jaundice (Gartner, 1994).

194. **(D)** Physiologic jaundice of the newborn is very common. Breast-feeding infants tend to have higher serum bilirubin concentrations in the early weeks of life with lower caloric intake seen as the critical factor (Newman & Maisels, 1992). In light of the absence of other risk factors, it would be appropriate to encourage frequent, effective breast-feeding, examine the blood for hematocrit, hemoglobin, and peripheral smear, and repeat the bilirubin the following day.

195. **(B)** Hemolytic disease in the newborn is a risk factor in developing high serum bilirubin concentrations. Useful laboratory evaluations are a hematocrit and hemoglobin to look for anemia, a blood smear for erythrocyte morphology, and ABO, Rh, and Coombs' testing on cord blood in those infants whose mothers are Rh-negative. The reticulocyte count is of little value in the newborn unless significant anemia is detected (Gartner, 1994).

196. **(B)** Physiologic jaundice is defined as clinical jaundice over 24 hours of age, with a total bilirubin that rises by < 5 mg/dL. It is characterized by a peak at 3–5 days with a total bilirubin level that is < 15 mg/dL and clinical jaundice that resolves by 1 week in the term and 2 weeks in the preterm infant (Rosenberg & Thilo, 1997). Therefore, the infant in this case has jaundice that is within physiologic parameters.

197. **(A)** Adequate caloric intake helps to diminish the risk of high serum bilirubin concentrations. Therefore, it is important to assure adequacy of caloric intake in infants who are breast-feeding. Signs of inadequate breast milk intake are weight loss > 8–10% from birth weight, < 6 wet diapers per day, < 4 stools per day, with a lesser frequency of nursing (Rosenberg & Thilo, 1997).

198. **(D)** Phototherapy has been found to be an effective treatment in reducing serum bilirubin levels (Gartner, 1994). The American Academy of Pediatrics (AAP) committee guidelines on the management of jaundice in a healthy, term neonate indicate bilirubin levels that warrant phototherapy treatment (AAP, 1994).

199. **(D)** Transmission of HIV occurs predominantly from mother to infant either during pregnancy, during delivery, or through breast-feeding in 85–90% of children with AIDS (Larson, 1995). Only 13–40% of children born to HIV-infected women become infected by the virus, although the factors contributing to this transmission are not well defined. Among adolescents, heterosexual transmission is the most common mode of transmission of the AIDS virus (Rand & Meyers, 1993).

200. **(B)** All HIV-infected children should receive their routine vaccinations. Recommended modifications include: (1) eliminating all live virus vaccines except for measles, mumps, and rubella (MMR) because of the potential for severe measles; (2) routine administration of *Haemophilus influenzae* type B (Hib), hepatitis B, diphtheria, pertussis, and tetanus (DPT) immunizations; (3) administration of influenza vaccine after 6 months of age; (4) administration of pneumococcal polysaccharide vaccine after 24 months of age; and (5) use of an inactive poliovirus vaccine, because the vaccine strain of polio can revert to a virulent strain in the gastrointestinal tract (Rand & Meyers, 1993). Varicella-zoster virus vaccine is contraindicated in these individuals.

201. **(A)** The clinical manifestations of HIV infection are often variable in children. Unusual or severe forms of common pediatric illnesses may occur, such as otitis, fevers, thrush, diarrhea, and pneumonia. Some infants who are infected perinatally may develop severe illnesses such as *Pneumocystis carinii*. Kaposi's sarcoma, a common condition in adults infected with the AIDS virus, is rare in children with AIDS (Larson & Bechtel, 1995).

202. **(A)** *Pneumocystis carinii* is the most common life-threatening, opportunistic infection of children with HIV infection. Therefore, children infected with the AIDS virus should receive prophylactic therapy for *P. carinii* with trimethoprim-sulfamethoxazole (TMP-SMZ). Fever, tachypnea, and hypoxia are common presenting signs of *P. carinii.* Although infections are common complications in HIV-infected children, routine prophylaxis against them are not currently recommended (Rand & Meyers, 1993).

203. **(C)** HIV transmission and the care of HIV-infected individuals are still often misunderstood, leaving individuals and families feeling stigmatized. Children who are infected require stable living conditions where their psychosocial, emotional, physical, and educational needs are met. If well enough, HIV-infected children should attend school and may attend day care if necessary. Measures should be taken to minimize exposure of the HIV-infected child to contagious illness. Universal precautions should be applied in the care of all children to maximize protection to all individuals (Larson & Bechtel, 1995; Rand & Meyers, 1993).

204. **(C)** The prevention of HIV infection in children should begin with the prevention of infection in women of childbearing age, such as offering HIV testing to all pregnant women. Zidovudine, an antiretroviral therapy, has been found to reduce the risk of perinatal transmission and is recommended in the management of all pregnant, HIV-infected women [Morbidity, Mortality Weekly Reports (MMWR), 1994].

205. **(A)** The complete blood count (CBC) with differential is the most helpful initial test in the diagnosis of acute lymphoblastic leukemia (ALL). The disease commonly presents with anemia and thrombocytopenia. The white blood count (WBC) is usually low or normal, hemoglobin (Hgb) counts are low, platelet counts are decreased, and neutropenia is common (Poplack & Reaman, 1988). Choice B is of normal lab values, and in choice C the blood count is normal except for a low platelet count, which may be indicative of idiopathic thrombocytopenia purpura (ITP).

206. **(C)** Acute lymphoblastic leukemia (ALL) is the most common form of malignancy in

childhood. Approximately 2500 cases per year are diagnosed in the United States. The peak incidence occurs at 4 years of age, with a range of 2–10 years. It is seen twice as commonly in whites as in nonwhites. The presenting symptoms of ALL reflect the degree of bone marrow infiltration by leukemic lymphoblasts. Common initial signs and symptoms are bone pain, hepatosplenomegaly, intermittent fevers, and pallor and fatigue. Although anorexia is common, significant weight loss is rare (Poplack & Reaman, 1988; Albano et al., 1997)

207. **(D)** Patients receiving chemotherapy for ALL should be prophylaxed against *Pneumocystis carinii* with trimethoprim-sulfamethoxazole, given on two to three consecutive days per week, twice a day (Albano et al., 1997). If left untreated, infection with *Pneumocystis carinii* is usually fatal.

208. **(B)** Infection is recognized as the major cause of morbidity and mortality in children with ALL, with the lung as the most common site of serious infection (Albano & Pizzo, 1988). It is therefore important to evaluate the febrile child with leukemia quickly and thoroughly in an effort to reduce the risk to the individual.

209. **(D)** Brain tumors are the most common form of malignant solid tumors in children and account for approximately 1700 new cases per year in the United States (Cohen & Garvin, 1996). Although prognoses for some cancers have improved, cancer is second only to accidents as the leading cause of death in children. Presenting signs and symptoms are related to the age of the child and location of the tumor; however, seizures are not the most common presenting symptoms. Astrocytoma is the most common type of brain tumor in children (Albano et al., 1997).

210. **(C)** Brain tumors in children may produce increased intracranial pressure (IICP), which leads to "classic" brain tumor symptoms, such as headache that is present on arising, relieved by vomiting without nausea, and lessening during the day (Albano et al., 1997). In infants,

IICP may present when there is impairment of the upward gaze and downward deviation of the eyes, known as "sun-setting sign."

211. **(B)** Both neuroblastoma and Wilms' tumor are the most common forms of abdominal tumors in children. Wilms' tumor arises from the kidney, and children between 2 and 5 years are most commonly affected. Most children present with an enlarged abdomen or with an abdominal mass that is often asymptomatic (Albano et al., 1997).

212. **(A)** Retinoblastoma is the most common intraocular tumor in children, with the majority of cases occurring before age 5 years. Sixty percent of children with retinoblastoma present with leukocoria (white pupillary reflex); however, strabismus is seen in 20% of cases. The child with suspected retinoblastoma must have a detailed ophthalmologic exam and a CT scan to evaluate the extent of the tumor infiltration (Albano et al., 1997).

213. **(D)** Aside from medical complications, children with cancer have to cope with a myriad of psychosocial issues. These include school problems related to long-term radiation therapy, which in turn can lead to poor self-esteem and peer relationship difficulties; and adverse effects on family relationships as well as the financial burden that a long-term illness places on individuals and their families (Carter, Thompson, & Simone, 1991).

214. **(C)** Children who are between the ages of 1 and 3 years are at greatest risk of lead poisoning, because this is the age of greatest hand-to-mouth activity (Schonfeld, 1994).

215. **(C)** In 1991, the CDC recommended universal blood lead screening for all children 6–72 months based on risk factors for exposure. Using this paradigm, otherwise asymptomatic children at low risk for lead exposure should be screened at 12 and 24 months of age. Asymptomatic children who have risk factors identified should be screened at 6 months and again at 12 months of age (Overby, 1996; CDC, 1991).

216. **(D)** The CDC guidelines of 1991 set the threshold of lead poisoning prevention at 10 μg/dL. While a blood lead level of 15 μg/dL requires education, nutrition counseling, and retesting, levels > 20 require medical evaluation and may require treatment and follow-up. Although the child with lead poisoning is often asymptomatic, any child with symptoms of acute lead poisoning should be evaluated thoroughly (Overby, 1996).

217. **(A)** Education about lead poisoning prevention is critical to eliminating this significant health problem in children. Although the major source of exposure for children is lead-based paint, other sources of lead exposure include paint dust, soil, water, occupational exposure as well as many lesser-known sources such as colored newsprint (Schonfeld, 1994).

218. **(D)** Children who experience pica or have unexplained seizures, neurologic symptoms, developmental delay, or abdominal pain should have laboratory evaluation for lead toxicity regardless of their age or risk factors (Overby, 1996).

219. **(C)** Iron deficiency anemia is the leading cause of anemia among infants and children in the United States (Kline, 1996). Although the incidence has declined in recent years due to the iron supplementation of infant formula and food products, it still remains prevalent in children under 2 years of age, especially with a history of excessive milk intake. Even large amounts of milk contain negligible amounts of iron. Nutritional iron deficiency anemia can be complicated by stool blood loss secondary to the effect of heat-labile cow's milk protein on intestinal mucosa. Therefore, the child must rely on other dietary sources of iron. Green leafy vegetables and red meat are both good sources of iron in this child's diet.

220. **(A)** When evaluating children with suspected anemia, it is important to investigate whether the child has a family history significant for anemia, jaundice, or gallstones. In addition, racial and ethnic backgrounds are also significant factors. A child of Mediterranean origin is at risk of developing thalassemia syndromes, and G6PD deficiency is more likely among Africans, Greeks, Filipinos, Sardinians, and Jews. Hemoglobin S and C are more common in the black population; the alpha-thalassemia trait is more common among blacks and Asians (Oski, 1993).

221. **(D)** In addition to the data collected through a detailed history and physical exam, lab interpretation is an essential component in the initial assessment of the child with suspected anemia. Diagnostic features of iron deficiency anemia include a hemoglobin and hematocrit > 2 standard deviations (SD) below normal for that child's age, red blood cell (RBC) size—assessed by mean corpuscular volume (MCV)—that is > 2 SD below mean for that child's age, and RBCs that are small and pale on peripheral smear. If a young child's anemia is thought to be due to immune causes, a Coombs test is warranted. A child with jaundice accompanied by hemolytic disease or liver pathology should be evaluated with liver function tests (LFT's) and bilirubin studies (Kline, 1996).

222. **(A)** Common features of mild iron deficiency anemia (IDA) include pallor, easy fatigability, irritability, and anorexia (Bushnell, 1992). A child who is otherwise healthy, but who has a slow and insidious onset may tolerate anemia well, manifesting few symptoms. More severe cases of anemia may cause an increase in cardiac output with resultant congestive heart failure because of the high output state. These clients may experience tachycardia and tachypnea. Iron deficiency anemia may also effect a child's neurologic and intellectual function (Oski, 1993).

223. **(C)** The differential diagnosis of childhood anemias is based on red blood cell (RBC) size. Microcytic hypochromic anemias, such as iron deficiency anemia, have low values of mean corpuscular volume (MCV). Macrocytic anemias, such as folate deficiency, have high values of MCV and show large RBCs on smears. Anemias that originate from intrinsic RBC defects, such as sickle cell disease (SCD), are normochromic and normocytic, with normal MCV values. Chronic infection, such as hepatitis followed by aplastic anemia, would be manifested by a decreased RBC production and normal MCV values (Schwartz, 1996).

224. **(B)** The appropriate treatment for iron deficiency anemia is 4–6 mg/kg/day of elemental iron divided into 3 daily doses. Treatment should continue for 3 months; 1 month to correct the anemia and 2 additional months to replenish iron stores. Checking a reticulocyte count in 4–7 days or a hematocrit–hemoglobin in 3–4 weeks is recommended to confirm the diagnosis. To prevent a recurrence of the problem, dietary counseling regarding iron-containing foods and reducing milk intake is also necessary.

Cardiovascular

CASES AND QUESTIONS

Questions 225–228

Raymond is a 4-year-old, healthy boy with normal growth and development who presents to his PNP for a routine physical. Upon auscultation, the PNP notes a grade 2/6, musical, short systolic murmur, which is best heard at the left lower sternal border; it does not radiate to the axillary region or back. The murmur is somewhat louder in the supine position. Both heart sounds are audible, and the second heart sound is occasionally split.

225. The most likely diagnosis of this murmur is

   (A) Atrial septal defect (ASD)
   (B) Small ventricular septal defect (VSD)
   (C) Still's murmur
   (D) Cervical venous hum

226. The management of this patient by the PNP should include

   (A) An echocardiogram to rule out significant heart disease
   (B) Subacute bacterial endocarditis (SBE) prophylaxis for all dental and surgical procedures
   (C) Follow-up every 4 months to check heart rate, blood pressure, pulses, and weight gain
   (D) None of the above

227. What factor(s) would increase the likelihood that Raymond's murmur requires more immediate referral to a pediatric cardiologist for evaluation?

   (A) Raymond has a history of mild gastro-esophageal reflux (GER) as an infant.
   (B) Raymond's mother was diagnosed with a flow murmur during her pregnancy with Raymond.
   (C) Raymond has trisomy 21.
   (D) All of the above.

228. Which of the following statements about all children with murmurs is *true?*

   (A) A screening EKG and CXR is never necessary.
   (B) 50% of all children at some point in childhood will have an innocent murmur.
   (C) All children should be referred to a pediatric cardiologist before their first dental exam.
   (D) One out of 50 patients will be diagnosed with some form of congenital heart disease.

Questions 229–232

Shakira is a 2½-year-old child whose past medical history includes several pneumonias and poor growth in the first 6 months of life. She presents for a routine check-up; her weight and height are at the 50th percentile. Her mother worries that Shakira looks "pale."

229. Shakira's blood pressure in her right leg is 100/62, and 88/58 in her right arm. Her pulses are palpable and equal. The PNP should

(A) Continue with the exam; her blood pressures are within normal range
(B) Consider coarctation of the aorta as a likely diagnosis and refer Shakira to a pediatric cardiologist
(C) Obtain an O_2 saturation in Shakira's lower exremity and compare it with an O_2 saturation in the upper extremity
(D) Recheck Shakira's blood pressures in 2 weeks

230. Upon physical exam, Shakira's lungs are clear to auscultation, and her abdomen is soft and without organomegaly. On cardiac exam, she has a regular rate and rhythym and no murmur. Her first and second heart sounds are audible, and the second heart sound is widely split and fixed throughout inspiration and expiration. No thrill is palpated. The PNP should

(A) Reassure Shakira's parents that her cardiac exam is normal, since she has no murmur
(B) Consider atrial septal defect (ASD) as a possible diagnosis and refer her to a pediatric cardiologist
(C) Refer Shakira to a cardiologist only if she contines to have frequent pneumonia
(D) Draw a complete blood count (CBC); if the hemoglobin and hematocrit are normal, no cardiac follow-up is necessary

231. Which of the following statements is *true* about children with atrial septal defects (ASD)?

(A) Most children with ASD are symptomatic with fatiue and failure to gain weight.
(B) Subacute bacterial endocarditis (SBE) prophylaxis with dental and surgical procedures is required in children with uncomplicated secundum ASD.
(C) Pulmonary vascular disease may develop in adulthood if lesions are not surgically repaired.
(D) Almost all large ASDs will close on their own by 5 years of age.

232. Which of the following statements about pediatric cardiovascular disorders is *true*?

(A) The presence of a thrill usually signifies pathologic heart disease.
(B) All children with congenital heart disease must be on SBE prophylaxis.
(C) ASDs are the most common congenital heart defect.
(D) Over 80% of children with trisomy 21 (Down syndrome) have some type of congenital heart disease.

Questions 233–236

Martin is a 2-week-old boy, born at 32 weeks' gestation to a 38-year-old G8, P8 mother. His mother's pregnancy was relatively benign, and she was on Dilantin for a childhood seizure disorder. Martin was born by emergency cesarean section with a birth weight of 2.8 kg, and Apgar scores of 6 at 1 minute, and 7 at 5 minutes. He required no intubation and was discharged after 12 days with good weight gain and an audible murmur on his discharge exam. One of Martin's older brothers had been diagnosed with critical pulmonary stenosis at birth, and died at 5 days of age.

233. Which of the following factors predisposes Martin to a higher possibility of having some type of congenital heart disease?

(A) Prematurity at 32 weeks of age
(B) Sibling with a history of congenital heart disease
(C) Maternal use of Dilantin to control her seizure disorder
(D) All of the above

234. Which of the following murmurs is common during infancy and is considered to be an innocent murmur?

(A) Peripheral pulmonary stenosis
(B) Cervical venous hum
(C) Patent ductus arteriosus
(D) Small muscular ventricular septal defect

235. Martin is diagnosed with a ventricular septal defect (VSD) and is followed by a pediatric cardiologist regularly. His PNP should be alarmed by all the following EXCEPT

    (A) Martin's weight drops significantly over a short period of time.
    (B) Martin takes more that 45 minutes to drink 4 oz.
    (C) Martin develops frequent respiratory tract infections.
    (D) Martin has a palpable liver edge.

236. All of the following statements are true of children with VSD EXCEPT

    (A) VSD murmur is not always associated with a palpable thrill.
    (B) SBE prophylaxis is needed before surgical repair.
    (C) VSDs can become larger as the child grows.
    (D) Spontaneous closure of small VSDs occurs over 60% of the time, and usually occurs during infancy.

Questions 237–239

Ronnie is a previously healthy 4-year-old male with a history of eczema and asthma, who presents to his PNP for a well-child exam. His weight and height are at the 50th percentile. His mother reports that Ronnie has been complaining that his "heart hurts" for the last 3 days. He has otherwise been active and eating well, and he has had no fever, nausea, vomiting, or diarrhea. On auscultatory exam, the PNP notes an irregular heart beat but no wheezing. There is no murmur, and his heart rate is 80 beats per minute.

237. What next step should the PNP take in determining the type of rhythm heard?

    (A) It can be assumed that Ronnie has a sinus tachycardia since no murmur is present.
    (B) A 12-lead EKG should be performed.
    (C) Ronnie must be referred to a pediatric cardiologist before a rhythm disturbance can be determined.
    (D) Ask Ronnie to breathe deeply and rapidly for 15 seconds: If the heart rate speeds up with this manuever, it can be assumed that Ronnie has a sinus arrhythmia.

238. A 12-lead EKG reveals premature ventricular contractions with every other beat. Ronnie is playful and active and does not complain of chest pain. His blood pressure is 90/56. The next step the PNP should take in this patient's management is

    (A) Prescribe acetaminophen for Ronnie's chest pain and follow up with him in 1 year.
    (B) Refer him to a pediatric cardiologist.
    (C) Teach Ronnie's mother how to take a pulse, and have her call if his heart rate is faster than 120 beats per minute.
    (D) Reassure Ronnie's mother that isolated premature beats can be normal.

239. All the following statements about supraventricular tachycardia (SVT) are true EXCEPT

    (A) SVT frequently presents in infancy with signs and symptoms of congestive heart failure.
    (B) It only takes 1–2 hours of continuous SVT for signs and symptoms of congestive heart failure to become apparent.
    (C) Applying pressure to the eyeball is contraindicated in the treatment of SVT due to the risk of retinal detachment.
    (D) The risk of suddent death caused by SVT is rare in children with structurally normal hearts.

Questions 240–243

Katarina is a 2-month-old infant who was born by NSVD at 40 weeks. She is growing and eating well, and is developmentally appropriate for age. On physical exam, the PNP notes a grade 1–2/6 short murmur that is audible at the axilla and the back bilaterally and equally. Katarina's heart rate is approximately 120 beats per minute. Her lungs are clear, and her abdomen is soft and without organomegaly. Her skin is warm and pink and her pulses are equal in all four extremities.

240. How best may the PNP determine whether the murmur is systolic or diastolic in nature?

  (A) Wait until the 4- or 6-month visit when the heart rate has slowed, since it is too difficult to determine in a tachycardic infant.
  (B) A diastolic murmur can be automatically ruled out because Katarina does not have a palpable thrill.
  (C) Palpate the brachial pulse with auscultation: If the murmur coincides with a palpable pulse, the murmur must be systolic.
  (D) Since there is no audible click and the patient appears healthy, a systolic murmur can be assumed.

241. The most likely diagnosis of this murmur is

  (A) Coarctation of the aorta
  (B) Peripheral pulmonary stenosis
  (C) Still's murmur
  (D) Atrial septal defect

242. The management of this patient by the PNP should include:

  (A) Immediate referral to a pediatric cardiologist since all murmurs that radiate to the back are pathologic

  (B) Documenting the murmur without sharing the physical findings with the parents yet to avoid needless parental anxiety
  (C) Seeing the patient more frequently than normal and asking the family to notify you in case of cyanosis or respiratory distress
  (D) Documenting the findings and referring the patient only if she is symptomatic or if the murmur persists beyond 6 months of age

243. All the following physical findings are usually associated with pathologic murmurs EXCEPT

  (A) A grade 1/6 soft, systolic ejection murmur
  (B) Continuous murmur, heard throughout systole and diastole
  (C) Systolic ejection click
  (D) A grade 1/6 diastolic murmur

ANSWERS AND RATIONALES

225.   (C) Still's murmur is commonly heard in children with an otherwise normal physical exam and no symptomatology. The murmur is classically a musical type of murmur that is heard at the left sternal border with normal heart sounds and with no significant radiation. The murmur can sometimes be louder in the supine position (Fyler, 1992; Allen, Golinko, & Williams, 1994).

226.   (D) Children with Still's murmur need no further workup because the murmur is an innocent murmur. The parents need only be reassured that their child is healthy and does not need any specific activity restrictions. SBE prophylaxis is never needed for innocent murmurs (Fyler, 1992).

227.   (C) Because children with trisomy 21 (Down syndrome) have a 40% chance of having congenital heart disease, it is imperative that those children with murmurs be referred to a pediatric cardiologist for evaluation, even if the physical findings are consistent with an innocent murmur (Allen et al., 1994; Fyler, 1992; Hazinski, 1992).

228.   (B) Fifty percent of all children at some point in childhood will have an innocent murmur. Therefore, those patients with innocent murmurs do not always need to be evaluated by a pediatric cardiologist. The prevalence of congenital heart disease has been constant over time, with an incidence of between 0.4 and 1% in the general population (Fyler, 1992).

229.   (A) Coarctation of the aorta should be suspected when the lower extremitiy blood pressures are *lower* than the upper extremity blood pressures. The systolic pressure in the femoral artery can normally be up to 20 mm Hg higher than in the arm. Therefore, blood pressures that are higher in the lower extremities are generally not worrisome. However, if upper extremity blood pressures are only slightly higher than the lower extremity blood pressures, the clinician should be alerted, as this may represent a significant difference (Fyler, 1992). Blood pressures should be reassessed in the supine position for the most accurate four extremity blood pressures. Using the correct size cuff is critical to obtaining accurate readings. A cuff too small may falsely elevate a blood pressure reading, while a cuff too large may falsely give a lower reading (McEvoy, 1981).

230.   (B) Auscultatory findings in children with atrial septal defect (ASD) include a second heart sound that is widely split, with the splitting varying little with respirations. The wide split results from a delayed closure of the pulmonary valve, as a result of emptying an overloaded right ventricle. In rare cases, there may be no systolic murmur at all (Fyler, 1992). In cases of cyanotic heart disease, most children are polycythemic rather than anemic.

231.   (C) The main reason to close ASDs is to prevent pulmonary vascular disease in adulthood. Antimicrobial prophylaxis is not necessary for children with uncomplicated secundum atrial septal defects (Fyler, 1992).

232. **(A)** The palpation of a thrill is *never* associated with functional murmurs. Therefore, patients with palpable thrills should referred to a pediatric cardiologist for evaluation to rule out pathologic heart disease (McEvoy, 1981). Atrial septal defects are responsible for approximately 12% of all congenital heart lesions (Hazinski, 1992).

233. **(D)** Premature infants are at risk for having patent ductus arteriosus. The risk of recurrence of congenital heart disease to a family with one affected child is thought to be between 1 and 3% or greater with some types of defects (Fyler, 1992; Allen et al., 1994). Maternal use of some drugs during pregnancy, including Dilantin, is associated with different types of congenital heart defects (Allen et al., 1994).

234. **(A)** Peripheral pulmonary stenosis (PPS), also known as a pulmonary flow murmur, is a type of innocent murmur that is heard in systole and transmits to the axillae and back bilaterally (Allen et al., 1994). A cervical venous hum is an innocent murmur but is not typically heard until childhood (Fyler, 1992).

235. **(D)** A palpable liver edge can be a normal finding in most infants. Poor growth, difficulty with eating, and frequent respiratory tract infections are worrisome signs in a patient diagnosed with a ventricular septal defect and can represent signs of congestive heart failure (Fyler, 1992).

236. **(C)** Ventricular defects do not get bigger, only smaller (Fyler, 1992).

237. **(B)** The cornerstone in the diagnosis of arrythmias is the use of an EKG machine (Robinson, Anisman, & Eshaghpour, 1996). Rate, not rhythm, can be determined by auscultation.

238. **(B)** Although Ronnie is playful and active, and not complaining of chest pain at the time of the EKG, his frequency of premature contractions and history of chest pain should alert the clinician to make a referral to a pediatric cardiologist. Ventricular ectopy on a routine EKG can be a manifestation of an underlying arrhythmia. Asymptomatic patients with isolated premature ventricular contractions and a normal heart do not require treatment (Fyler, 1992).

239. **(B)** It usually takes more than 24 hours of continuous supraventricular tachycardia (SVT) for signs and symptoms of congestive heart failure to become apparent (Robinson et al., 1996).

240. **(C)** Most infants are tachycardic, making it difficult to assess whether the audible murmur is systolic or diastolic. The simple manuever of palpating the pulse while auscultating the murmur makes the assessment somewhat easier (Allen et al., 1994).

241. **(B)** Peripheral pulmonary stenosis (PPS) is a type of innocent murmur that is heard in systole and transmits to the axillary region and back bilaterally. This murmur usually disappears by 6 months of age (Fyler, 1992).

242. **(D)** Peripheral pulmonary stenosis is an innocent murmur that does not warrant referral to a pediatric cardiologist unless the patient has other worrisome signs or symptoms, or if the murmur persists beyond 6 months (Burton & Cabalka, 1994).

243. **(A)** A grade 1/6 soft systolic ejection murmur can often be associated with an innocent murmur. Continuous murmurs *can* be associated with pathologic heart disease, but not exclusively. Cervical venous hum, for example, is a type of innocent murmur that is continuous throughout systole and diastole. Any diastolic murmur is abnormal, and a systolic ejection click is indicative of an abnormal aortic or pulmonary valve (Fyler, 1992).

Respiratory

CASES AND QUESTIONS

Questions 244–247

Jasmine is a 2-year-old female who has had two previous episodes of wheezing since age 12 months. She has a 4-year-old male sibling with asthma. She has never required hospitalization. Only one of her previous exacerbations required use of prednisolone. Her current medications are cromolyn sodium (Intal) bid and albuterol (Ventolin) via nebulizer only with acute exacerbations of wheezing. To date, her asthma triggers have been viral upper respiratory infections.

244. All the following statements are true about asthma in childhood EXCEPT

    (A) It is the most common chronic illness in childhood.
    (B) It occurs in equal numbers among males and females.
    (C) Often there is a family history of asthma.
    (D) Often there is an individual or family history of atopy.

245. Asthma, regardless of its severity, is defined as

    (A) An acute hyperresponsive disease of the airways
    (B) An acute allergic disease of the airways
    (C) A chronic allergic disease of the airways
    (D) A chronic inflammatory disease of the airways

246. Factors that increase the risk of asthma include

    (A) History of prematurity
    (B) Inner-city residence
    (C) Male gender
    (D) All of the above

247. The first step in asthma control is

    (A) Avoiding triggers
    (B) Pharmacologic agents
    (C) Nutritional supplementation
    (D) Breathing exercises

Questions 248–252

Jasmine presents today to your office with a 2-day history of upper respiratory infection with clear rhinorrhea and loose cough. Her temperature is 37.2°C (99°F) rectally, RR 38/min with mild intercostal retractions, no flaring, no grunting, apical pulse 120. Her chest is tight with diffuse expiratory wheezes bilaterally. Her O_2 saturation by pulse oximetry is 93% on room air. Her HEENT examination is normal. She is well hydrated. She last received albuterol 0.3 cc via nebulizer 1½ hours prior to this visit.

248. Clinical findings that might be consistent with asthma in a young child include all of the following EXCEPT

    (A) Increased expiratory flow
    (B) Exercise intolerance
    (C) Wheezing
    (D) Frequent cough

249. All the following are clinical signs of respiratory distress in children EXCEPT

    (A) Mouth breathing
    (B) Intercostal retractions
    (C) Tachypnea
    (D) Nasal flaring

250. Components of acute asthma attack include all of the following EXCEPT

    (A) Laryngeal edema
    (B) Mucus hypersecretion
    (C) Bronchospasm
    (D) Inflammation of airway mucosa

251. Symptoms of asthma are usually precipitated by recognizable triggers such as

    1. Warm air
    2. Allergens and pollutants
    3. Viral infections
    4. Exercise
        (A) 1 and 2
        (B) 2 and 4
        (C) 2, 3, 4
        (D) All of the above

252. The most common preventable asthma trigger in children is

    (A) Seasonal allergies
    (B) Household molds
    (C) Passive cigarette smoke
    (D) Dust mites

Questions 253–257

The PNP gives Jasmine an albuterol 0.3 cc nebulizer treatment in the office. Evaluation following this treatment shows a decrease in her intercostal retractions, decrease in RR to 30, and a rise in her O_2 saturation by pulse oximetry to 94% on room air. Breath sounds are clearer with improved aeration bilaterally. She continues to have scattered expiratory wheezes bilaterally. Jasmine receives a second Ventolin 0.3 cc nebulizer treatment. The PNP also decides to administer a dose of oral prednisolone (2 mg/kg) to Jasmine.

253. Role of oral prednisolone in an acute asthma exacerbation is

    (A) To provide prompt relief of bronchospasm
    (B) As an antiinflammatory agent, to speed recovery and prevent recurrence of exacerbation
    (C) To provide bronchodilation
    (D) All of the above

254. Jasmine's asthma patterns would most likely fall into which classification of asthma severity?

    (A) Mild intermittent asthma
    (B) Mild persistent asthma
    (C) Moderate persistent asthma
    (D) Severe persistent asthma

255. The pharmacologic agents used to treat asthma include medications used for long-term control and those used for quick rescue. Quick rescue asthma medications include which of the following?

    1. Short-acting beta-2-agonists
    2. Systemic corticosteroids
    3. Inhaled corticosteroids
    4. Mast-cell inhibitors
        (A) All of the above
        (B) 1 and 2
        (C) 3 and 4
        (D) 1, 2, 4

256. Which of the following steps would be included in Jasmine's at-home asthma management plan?

    (A) Continue to use cromolyn daily for long-term control.
    (B) Use albuterol for relief of acute symptoms and before exposure to known allergens.
    (C) Review basic asthma education and action plans with family.
    (D) All of the above.

257. Current recommendation is for patients with moderate to severe asthma to learn to monitor their peak flow with a peak flow meter at home. All the following statements are *true* about peak flow monitoring EXCEPT

    (A) Peak flow monitoring can help promote self-management and compliance with pharmacologic regime.
    (B) Peak flow monitoring monitors a child's response to pharmacologic intervention.
    (C) Peak flow monitoring does not help identify asthma triggers.
    (D) Peak flow monitoring can predict acute asthma exacerbation.

Questions 258–261

Mark is a 6-month-old infant with a history of mild to moderate URI symptoms over the past 48 hours. The parent reports that Mark has been coughing frequently and "breathing really fast." He has been breast-feeding on his regular schedule without difficulty. He attends family day care 3 times a week. Mark is a full-term healthy infant with no history of underlying respiratory or cardiac disease. Physical examination reveals an infant with bilateral expiratory wheezes with mild crackles, copious clear nasal discharge, T 37.7 °C (100°F) rectally, and RR 48/min with an oxygen saturation of 96% on room air. He is well hydrated.

258. Which of the following respiratory conditions is the most likely cause of his cough and wheezing?

    (A) Asthma
    (B) Bronchiolitis
    (C) Foreign body aspiration
    (D) Pertussis

A chest x-ray is obtained, which reveals hyperinflation. Albuterol 0.5% solution, 0.15 mg/kg/dose in 2 mL normal saline is administered via mask/nebulizer with favorable results.

259. In bronchiolitis in infants, predictors of severe disease include all of the following EXCEPT

    (A) Chronologic age < 3 months or gestational age < 34 weeks
    (B) Respiratory rate > 70
    (C) Oxygen saturation < 95% on room air
    (D) Frequent cough

260. The principal single cause of bronchiolitis is

    (A) *Haemophilus influenzae*
    (B) Respiratory syncytial virus (RSV)
    (C) Pneumococcus
    (D) Parainfluenza virus

261. Outpatient management for Mark may include all the following EXCEPT

    (A) Continuous humidified oxygen at home until clinically improved
    (B) Adequate oral fluid intake
    (C) Cool-mist therapy
    (D) Careful at-home observation for signs of increased respiratory distress

Questions 262–266

Rachel is a 14-year-old, fully immunized female who presents to your clinic with complaints of a cough for almost 2 weeks. She has remained afebrile during the entire illness. The cough occurs day and night with mild URI symptoms. The cough has been persistent but not paroxysmal. There has been no vomiting. Today at school she was told of two confirmed cases of pertussis among members of her field hockey team.

262. Characteristics of pertussis may include all the following EXCEPT

    (A) Transmission requires contact with infected individuals.
    (B) Mortality is greatest in adolescents.
    (C) Morbidity is highest in children less than 5 years of age.
    (D) It can be divided into three stages: catarrhal, paroxysmal, convalescent.

263. The differential diagnosis of pertussis includes all the following EXCEPT

    (A) Acute bronchitis
    (B) Laryngotracheobronchitis
    (C) Pneumonia
    (D) Tuberculosis

264. Which of the following laboratory tests would be most appropriate to confirm the diagnosis of pertussis in this 14-year-old?

    (A) A serologic test for pertussis
    (B) Chest x-ray
    (C) Complete blood count with differential
    (D) A nasopharyngeal culture for pertussis

265. The recommended antibiotic treatment for a child with suspected pertussis would be

    (A) Doxycycline 2–4 mg/kg/day orally divided bid for 14 days
    (B) Amoxicillin 40 mg/kg/day orally divided tid for 14 days

(C) Cefixime 8 mg/kg/day orally qd for 14 days

(D) Erythromycin 40–50 mg/kg/day orally divided qid for 14 days

Rachel's 4-year-old sister has received four doses of acellular DTaP vaccine in infancy (fourth dose at age 18 months). She is healthy, afebrile, and currently asymptomatic.

266. The most appropriate management of this 4-year-old child would include which of the following?

(A) A culture of the nasopharynx for pertussis

(B) Administration of another dose of DTaP vaccine and antibiotic prophylaxis

(C) A serologic test for pertussis

(D) Administration of human pertussis immune globulin

Questions 267–270

Mariah is a 2-year-old female who presents today with fever of 38.8°C (102°F) rectally. Over the past several days she has had a mild URI with decreased appetite. Last evening she awoke with "noisy breathing" and cough. She is nontoxic appearing and nonstridorous in your office.

267. Which of the following would *not* be included in the differential diagnosis for upper airway obstructive disorders?

(A) Pertussis

(B) Bacterial tracheitis

(C) Laryngotracheobronchitis

(D) Epiglottitis

Mariah exhibits a hoarse, barking cough with RR 32/min. O_2 saturation is 97% on room air by pulse oximetry. Color is pink, and she is well hydrated. There are mild intercostal retractions. Immunizations are up to date.

268. Based on health history and PE, the most likely diagnosis for Mariah is

(A) Viral pneumonia

(B) Laryngotracheobronchitis

(C) Epiglottitis

(D) Pertussis

269. The most common viral pathogen associated with croup is

(A) Rhinovirus

(B) Parainfluenza virus

(C) Coxsackievirus

(D) Echovirus

270. The PNP recommends the following management for Mariah:

(A) Racemic epinephrine

(B) High-dose intramuscular dexamethasone

(C) Cool-mist therapy, oral hydration, antipyretics, and at-home observation

(D) Immediate referral to a local emergency room

Questions 271–273

Three-year-old Jeanine is brought to the local emergency room. You note an anxious, toxic-appearing child with audible stridor, drooling, and suprasternal retractions. Jeanine's father relates that a fever of 39.4°C (103°F) came on suddenly earlier today. It is questionable whether her immunizations are UTD.

271. You suspect that this patient has acute epiglottitis. All of the following statements about epiglottitis are true EXCEPT

(A) The most serious complication of epiglottitis is sudden airway obstruction.

(B) Epiglottitis is a true pediatric emergency.

(C) Vigorous examination of the posterior pharynx is necessary to confirm the diagnosis of epiglottitis.

(D) The majority of acute epiglottitis is caused by *Haemophilus influenzae* type B.

272. Acute epiglottitis differs from croup in all of the following ways EXCEPT

(A) Symptoms of epiglottitis include fever and drooling.

(B) The child with epiglottitis will appear toxic and anxious or show signs of respiratory distress.

(C) There is a slow onset of illness with epiglottitis.

(D) Antibiotics play an essential part in treatment of epiglottitis.

273. Immunization with which of the following vaccines has substantially reduced the incidence of life-threatening epiglottitis in the United States?

(A) Hib vaccine
(B) HBV vaccine
(C) HBIG vaccine
(D) MMR vaccine

Questions 274–279

Grant is a 20-month-old male with a 1-week history of URI. He attends day care full time. The parent reports that over the past several days Grant has had a low-grade fever of 37.7°C (100°F) rectally at bedtime. Additional findings include a wet cough and decreased appetite. Tonight he appears tired and has a fever of 38.8°C (102°F) rectally. Physical examination findings are significant for decreased breath sounds in the left upper lobe, no wheezing, with a RR of 24 breaths/min. HEENT exam is unremarkable. Chest x-ray reveals a small left upper lobe infiltrate.

274. The most common causative agent associated with pneumonia in Grant's age group is

(A) Viruses
(B) *Mycoplasma pneumoniae*
(C) Pneumococcus
(D) Chlamydia

275. The most common complication of pneumonia is

(A) Respiratory failure
(B) Dehydration
(C) Bacteremia
(D) Pleural effusion

276. Appropriate management of this nontoxic-appearing, febrile 20-month-old child with a lobar infiltrate would include which of the following?

(A) Supportive treatment (rest, antipyretics, and adequate hydration)

(B) No specific medical management necessary at this time

(C) Observation at home and reevaluation in 24 hours

(D) Supportive treatment, oral antibiotics, and reevaluation in 48 hours

277. Bacterial pneumonia is characterized by all of the following EXCEPT

(A) Fever
(B) Gradual onset
(C) Tachypnea
(D) Lethargy

278. Which of the following characteristics is associated with pneumonia due to *Mycoplasma pneumoniae?*

(A) The most common cause of pneumonia among children over 5 years of age
(B) Gradual onset with headache, fever, and malaise
(C) Nonproductive cough
(D) All of the above

279. The most common causative agent of bacterial pneumonia at every age beyond the newborn period is

(A) *Streptococcus aureus*
(B) Group B streptococcus
(C) *Haemophilus influenzae*
(D) None of the above

Questions 280–283

Juan is a 3-year-old who presents to your clinic with a cough for 1 month. The cough occurs day and night. Over-the-counter cough preparations have not relieved his symptoms. He has been afebrile with a normal appetite and normal activity level. He has no past medical history of allergic rhinitis or reactive airway disease. There is no recent history of URI or pharyngitis. No family members have cough, fever, or URI.

280. The differential diagnosis for chronic cough in a preschool-age child would include all of the following EXCEPT

(A) Viral upper respiratory infections
(B) Reactive airway disease

(C) Foreign body aspiration

(D) *Mycoplasma pneumoniae* infection

281. The most common cause of chronic cough in children is

(A) Pertussis

(B) Cough-variant asthma

(C) Sinusitis

(D) Passive cigarette smoke exposure

Juan is alert and nontoxic appearing. He has a persistent but nonparoxysmal cough and there is no respiratory distress. There are no retractions or use of accessory muscles. His respiratory rate is normal. His chest is entirely clear except for scattered expiratory wheezes in his right lower lobe. Growth and development parameters are entirely normal and there has been no recent travel.

282. The most likely cause of this child's chronic cough and wheeze is

(A) Foreign body aspiration

(B) Reactive airway disease

(C) Bronchiolitis

(D) Pneumonia

283. Which of the following diagnostic tests might be useful in evaluating this child's chronic cough?

(A) Pulse oximetry

(B) Inspiratory/expiratory chest x-ray

(C) Peak expiratory flow meter reading

(D) Upper GI series

ANSWERS AND RATIONALES

244. **(B)** Asthma is the most common chronic illness of childhood, affecting an estimated 4.8 million children. Childhood asthma is often associated with atopy and, like atopic conditions such as eczema, tends to run in families (Kemper, 1997; Centers for Disease Control, 1995).

245. **(D)** The *National Asthma Education and Prevention Program* of the National Heart, Lung and Blood Institute (1997) defines asthma as "a chronic inflammatory disorder of the airways in which many cells and cellular elements play a role, in particular, mast cells, eosinophils, T lymphocytes, macrophages, neutrophils, and epithelial cells. In susceptible individuals, this inflammation causes recurrent episodes of wheezing, breathlessness, chest tightness and coughing. These episodes are usually associated with widespread but variable airflow obstruction that is often reversible either spontaneously or with treatment. The inflammation also causes an associated increase in the existing bronchial hyperresponsiveness to a variety of stimuli." (p.3).

246. **(D)** Factors that may increase the risk of asthma in childhood include male gender, an individual or family history of atopy, race, birth history (bronchopulmonary dysplasia, prematurity), environment, and family history of asthma.

247. **(A)** Very few children have symptoms of asthma all the time. In most cases, symptoms are triggered on occasion by a variety of things such as exercise, viral upper respiratory illnesses, or environmental allergies. Therefore, the first step in asthma control is to identify a child's "triggers" and take steps to avoid and/or control them (Kemper, 1997).

248. **(A)** Wheezing, exercise intolerance, and frequent cough are all common clinical findings in children with asthma. In asthma, an individual will have decreased expiratory flow due to airflow obstruction secondary to airway edema, chronic mucous plug formation, and acute bronchoconstriction.

249. **(A)** Clinical signs of respiratory distress in children may include tachypnea, tachycardia, nasal flaring, use of accessory muscles (intercostal/substernal retractions), dyspnea, grunting, pallor, or possible cyanosis.

250. **(A)** Asthma manifests itself in a range of symptoms that are usually precipitated by recognizable triggers. Prior to becoming symptomatic, the airways become inflamed and mucus production increases. These inflammatory changes combine to limit airflow to and from the alveoli (bronchospasm, bronchoconstriction).

251. **(C)** Common asthma triggers in children include allergens, pollutants, viral upper respiratory infections, exercise, medications, foods, and stress. Exercise—especially in cold, dry air—triggers symptoms in nearly 90% of asthmatics (Kemper, 1997).

252. **(C)** The most common preventable asthma trigger in children is passive cigarette smoke. Parental smoking triggers asthma symptoms and slows recovery from exacerbations (Beeber, 1996; Kemper, 1997). Maternal smoking during pregnancy increase the risk for asthma and affects fetal lung development (Martinez, Cline, & Burrows, 1992; Kemper, 1997).

253. **(B)** Airway inflammation is present in almost all children with asthma, even when asthma symptoms are well controlled. Inhaled and systemic corticosteroids are antiinflammatory agents that decrease this inflammation, speed recovery and prevent recurrence of exacerbation. Therefore, antiinflammatory agents have become the cornerstone of asthma management (National Asthma Education and Prevention Program, 1997).

254. **(B)** Medications for asthma control are used in a stepwise fashion geared to the severity of the child's symptoms. Emphasis is placed on achieving and maintaining long-term control of asthma symptoms. Children such as Jasmine with mild persistent asthma are at step two, requiring daily antiinflammatory medications for long-term control and quick relief medications, such as a short-acting beta-2-agonist, for relief of acute symptoms. (See Figure A254 following answers to this section, pp. 87–90.)

255. **(D)** Quick relief medications, for rescue or relief of acute symptoms, include short-acting beta-2-agonists and systemic corticosteroids given in "short bursts." Mast-cell inhibitors may be used for both quick relief or rescue and long-term control of symptoms. Inhaled corticosteroids are used for long-term control of symptoms. (See Table A255 following answers to this section, pp. 91–93.)

256. **(D)** In addition to pharmacologic intervention geared to Jasmine's level of asthma severity, successful long-term management depends on education and cooperation between clinician, family, and child. A written action plan for self-management and asthma control should be reviewed at all visits. Families should be educated about the course of the disease, avoidance of known triggers, how to monitor symptoms, and how to use medications (National Asthma Education and Prevention Program, 1997).

257. **(C)** The *1997 Guidelines for the Diagnosis and Management of Asthma* from the National Asthma Education and Prevention Program recommends that patients with moderate to severe persistent asthma learn to monitor their peak flow and have a peak flow meter at home. Home peak flow measurements can provide an objective assessment of the severity of the child's asthma and response to medications, can help identify asthma triggers, and often can predict acute asthma exacerbation. (See Figure A257 following answers to this section, p. 94.)

258. **(B)** Bronchiolitis is a wheezing-associated illness in infants and young children that causes acute respiratory illness resulting in obstruction of small airways. Serious cases of bronchiolitis occur most commonly in infants younger than 1 year. Infants and young children usually present with a history of cough and rhinorrhea for 3–5 days. The cough becomes more frequent, accompanied by copious nasal secretions and often a history of decreased feedings. On chest auscultation, most infants and children have wheezing along with retractions, tachypnea, and crackles on inspiration. Fever is often low grade, but may be variable (see Table A258).

259. **(D)** Infants who appear "toxic," who have a chronologic age < 3 months or gestational age < 34 weeks, who have a respiratory rate of more than 70 bpm, and whose chest x-rays show atelectasis are likely to require hospitalization (Welliver & Welliver, 1993). The best single predictor of the need for hospitalization is an oxygen saturation < 95% on room air followed by a toxic appearance.

260. **(B)** Respiratory syncytial virus (RSV) is recognized as the major cause of bronchiolitis and serious lower respiratory infection in infants under age 1 year. RSV occurs worldwide

TABLE A258. COMPARISON OF FINDINGS IN LOWER RESPIRATORY TRACT INFECTIONS AND RESPIRATORY DISEASES

	Upper Respiratory Infection	Asthma	Bronchitis	Bronchiolitis	Atypical Pneumonia	Bacterial Pneumonia
History						
Cough	Yes	Frequent	Yes	Yes	Yes	Yes
Sudden onset	Yes	Frequent	Yes	Yes	Occasional	Yes
Upper respiratory infection prodrome	—	Frequent	Yes	Yes	Frequent	Occasional
Toxicity	No	No	No	Yes	Occasional	Yes
Fever	No	Low	Occasional, low	Low	Usually low	High
Sputum	Minimal, post-pharyngeal	Infrequently, modest	Copious, purulent	No	Modest	Copious, purulent
Seasonal	Yes	Often	No	Yes	No	No
Examination						
Tachypnea	No	Frequent	Occasional	Yes	Occasional	Yes
Retractions	No	Frequent	No	Yes	Frequent	Yes
Decreased breath sounds	No	Frequent	No	Frequent	No	Focal
Wheeze	No	Usual	Frequent	Yes	Frequent	No
Rales	No	Infrequent	No	Yes	Yes	Yes
Rhonchi	Upper airway	Frequent	Yes	No	No	No
Laboratory						
Hypoxemia	No	Frequent	No	Frequent	Occasional	Frequent
Leukocytosis	No	Occasional	No	Infrequent	Infrequent	Yes
Hyperinflation	No	Usual	No	Yes	Occasional	No
Atelectasis	No	Frequent	Infrequent	Frequent	Occasional	Infrequent
Infiltrate	No	Infrequent	No	Occasional	Yes	Yes
Effusion	No	No	No	No	*Mycoplasma*	Occasional

Reprinted with permission from Lapin, C.D., & Schramm, C.M. (1997). Lower respiratory tract infections. In A.J. Schwartz, N.J. Blum, & J.A. Fein, eds. Pediatric primary care: A problem-oriented approach *(3rd ed.). St. Louis: Mosby.*

in annual epidemics. Although parainfluenza virus infections are also associated with lower respiratory infections in infants and young children, their effect on the very young is not as dramatic (Hall, 1993).

261. **(A)** Uncomplicated RSV infection may be treated on an outpatient basis. Treatment consists of supportive measures such as increased oral fluids, humidification, and use of acetaminophen for fever and irritability. The infant or young child should be reevaluated within 24 hours. The use of albuterol remains a controversial issue in outpatient treatment of RSV infection (Klassen, 1997). In addition to the above, an evaluation of family resources and reliability is necessary to determine if the infant or child can be evaluated and treated on an outpatient basis.

262. **(B)** Pertussis, or whooping cough, is a highly communicable respiratory disease caused by *Bordetella pertussis*. Transmission occurs by close contact with respiratory secretions of patients with disease. Pertussis begins with mild upper respiratory symptoms (catarrhal stage), which can proceed to a severe paroxysmal cough (paroxysmal stage) with a gradual waning of symptoms (convalescent stage). The attack rate and severity of illness are greatest in premature infants and infants in the first year of life. Sixty percent of reported pertussis cases occur in children younger than age 5 years (American Academy of Pediatrics, 1997). Fully immunized adults and adolescents recently have been recognized as major sources of pertussis (American Academy of Pediatrics, 1997).

263. **(B)** Lower respiratory tract infections—including acute bronchitis, pneumonia, and tuberculosis—are included in the differential diagnosis of pertussis. Laryngotracheobronchitis, also known as croup, is a viral infection of the upper respiratory tract.

264. **(D)** No single laboratory test is useful in all stages of pertussis. Nasopharyngeal cultures are most likely to be positive during the catarrhal and early paroxysmal stages and are rarely found after the fourth week of illness. Nasopharyngeal cultures, therefore, should be obtained in a patient whose cough onset has been within the last 14 days.

265. **(D)** Pertussis symptoms may be ameliorated if antibiotic treatment is begun during the catarrhal stage. If antibiotics are begun later in the course of the disease, the period of contagion will be decreased, but the duration of the cough may not be decreased. The drug of choice is erythromycin 40–50 mg/kg/day orally in four divided doses for 14 days (maximum 2 g/day) (American Academy of Pediatrics, 1997).

266. **(B)** Erythromycin (40–50 mg/kg/day orally in four divided doses (maximum 2 g for 14 days) is recommended for all household contacts and other close contacts (day care, sports teams), irrespective of age and vaccination status. The immunization status of close contacts should also be assessed. The sibling in this case study, who has received four doses of DTaP, would receive a booster dose of DTaP unless a dose had been given within the last 3 years (American Academy of Pediatrics, 1997).

267. **(A)** Differential diagnoses would include epiglottitis, peritonsillar abscess, bacterial tracheitis, foreign body, retropharyngeal abscess, and angioedema (Table A267).

268. **(B)** Laryngotracheobronchitis ("croup") is the most common cause of acute stridor in young children. It is characterized by acute onset of inspiratory stridor, a "barking" cough, hoarseness, fever, and retractions with variable degrees of respiratory distress. Symptoms are usually preceded by an upper respiratory infection.

269. **(B)** Viral agents are responsible for the majority of cases of croup. The leading viral organisms are parainfluenza viruses followed by respiratory syncytial virus (RSV) and adenoviruses. Viral croup is common in children ages 6 months to 3 years and usually occurs in fall–winter.

270. **(C)** Mild-to-moderate croup can be managed on an outpatient basis with standard treatment such as cool-mist therapy, oral hydration, antipyretics, and close at-home observation. Corticosteroid use remains controversial; however, several sources indicate that a single dose of dexamethasone, in the range of 0.5–0.6 mg/kg IM, is reasonable as a therapeutic trial to prevent subsequent hospitalization in the child

TABLE A267. INFECTIOUS CAUSES OF UPPER AIRWAY OBSTRUCTION

Disease	Clinical Signs	Age	Season	Causes	Diagnosis and Therapy
Croup	Stridor, barking cough, mild fever, hoarseness, URI, worse at night	6 mo–3 yr	Late fall–winter	Parainfluenza (other viruses)	Cool mist, racemic epinephrine (IPPB), ± brief steroid use
Epiglottitis	Abrupt onset, toxic, anxious, high fever, drooling, dysphagia, rare cough	3–7 yr	None	*H. influenza* B	Direct visualization,[a] nasotracheal intubation, IV antibiotics, ICU admit
Retropharyngeal abscess	Acute pharyngitis, high fever, toxic, dysphagia, hyperextension of head, drooling	Variable	None	Group A strep, *S. aureus*, anaerobic bacteria	Visualization,[a] lateral neck x-rays, IV antibiotics, surgery
Bacterial tracheitis	Crouplike illness, high fever, toxic	< 6 yr	Late fall–winter	*S. aureus*	Visualization,[a] lateral neck x-ray, racemic epinephrine, IV antibiotics

IPPB = intermittent positive pressure breathing; URI = upper respiratory infection.

[a] Visualization should be performed by experienced personnel under controlled settings (usually in the PICU or under general anesthesia). The use of lateral neck x-rays is often helpful, but does not replace direct visualization, and they should not be obtained without the patient being observed by a physician capable of managing the airway in case of an abrupt obstruction.

Reprinted with permission from Kirchner, K., & Abman, S.H. (1997). Respiratory tract. In G.B. Merenstein, D.W. Kaplan, & A.A. Rosenberg, eds. Handbook of pediatrics (18th ed., p. 492). Stamford, CT: Appleton & Lange.

with moderate to severe croup (Geelhoed, 1997; Fleisher & Crain, 1996; Cruz, 1995). Nebulized racemic epinephrine is reserved and administered (in the EW) to the child with severe croup who will be hospitalized (Ruddy, 1993, 1994).

271. **(C)** Epiglottitis is a life-threatening bacterial infection of the epiglottis and surrounding structures. The most common causative agent is *H. influenzae.* It is a true pediatric emergency. When a child is suspected to have epiglottitis, the management plan is concentrated on making a conclusive diagnosis and instituting therapy before the onset of airway obstruction (Fleischer & Crain, 1996). All attempts to visualize the epiglottis must be avoided in the child with suspected epiglottitis as the examination could initiate airway obstruction (Table A267).

272. **(C)** Unlike croup, epiglottitis has an abrupt onset of fever, drooling, stridor, and respiratory distress. The child is toxic and very anxious appearing. Unlike in viral croup, antibiotics play an essential part in treatment of epiglottitis by eliminating the local bacterial infection and limiting its spread to other sites.

273. **(A)** Introduced in 1988, *H. influenzae* type B vaccine, given beginning at age 2 months, has resulted in a dramatic decrease in the number of children with invasive infections due to this organism. Therefore, epiglottitis has recently become relatively uncommon (American Academy of Pediatrics, 1997).

274. **(A)** After 2 months of age, viruses remain the most common cause of pneumonias. The most common viruses include RSV, adenoviruses, parainfluenza virus, and enterovirus. Between ages 2 months and 2 years, viruses and chlamydia are the most frequent causes of infection. *S. pneumoniae* is the predominant bacterial isolate at every age beyond the newborn period. *Mycoplasma pneumoniae* is the most common cause of pneumonia in children older than age 5 years.

275. **(B)** The majority of pneumonias resolve without consequence. Rarely, extensive pulmo-

nary involvement leads to respiratory compromise. The most common complication of pneumonia, especially in infants and young children, is dehydration.

276. **(D)** Most viral pneumonias resolve with supportive therapy such as adequate oral hydration and antipyretics. However, because of the limitations in obtaining sputum cultures for bacteria, it is safest to presume a bacterial etiology in a child with a lobar infiltrate, a pleural effusion, a temperature of 102°F (39°C) or signs of clinical toxicity (Fleisher & Crain, 1996). Therefore, the child in this case would be treated on an outpatient basis with oral antibiotic therapy, supportive therapy, and follow-up appointment in 48 hours.

277. **(B)** Bacterial pneumonia generally has an abrupt onset with fever, chills, and tachypnea. A cough is a common but nonspecific complaint. The young child may present with lethargy and/or decreased appetite. Viral pneumonia has a gradual onset with cough, low-grade fever, and coryza.

278. **(D)** Mycoplasmal pneumonia is the most common cause of pneumonia in children age 5 years and over. The pneumonia has a gradual onset with fever and malaise that proceeds within 5 days to headache, sore throat, and nonproductive cough.

279. **(D)** In the newborn period, group B streptococcus and gram-negative bacilli cause the majority of bacterial pneumonias. The most common causative agent of bacterial pneumonia at every age beyond the newborn period is *Streptococcus pneumoniae.*

280. **(D)** Viral upper respiratory infections, reactive airway disease, and foreign body aspiration would all be differential diagnoses in cases of chronic cough in preschool-age children. *Mycoplasma pneumoniae* is the most common causative agent in pneumonias in children age 5 years to young adult (Table A258).

281. **(B)** Cough-variant asthma, often in the absence of wheezing, is the most common cause

of chronic cough in children (Rosenstein & Fosarelli, 1997). It may be precipitated by viral illness, exercise, cold air, pollutants (such as passive cigarette smoke), and allergens.

282.   **(A)** Clinicians should always consider foreign body aspiration in the differential diagnosis of chronic cough in a preschool-age child. Typically, this cough occurs day and night, has an acute onset, and is associated with unilateral wheezing or decreased respirations on the affected side. Foreign body aspiration may initially go unsuspected if there was no witnessed episode of choking or coughing.

283.   **(B)** When there is a suspected foreign body aspiration, air trapping on the affected side can be identified by one of the following: fluoroscopy, lateral decubitus chest x-ray, inspiratory/expiratory chest x-ray, or bronchoscopy (Rojas, O'Connell, & Sachs, 1991).

Stepwise Approach for Managing Infants and Young Children (5 Years of Age and Younger) With Acute or Chronic Asthma Symptoms

	Long-Term Control	Quick Relief
STEP 4 **Severe** **Persistent**	■ Daily antiinflammatory medicine – High-dose inhaled corticosteroid with spacer/holding chamber and face mask – If needed, add systemic corticosteroids 2 mg/kg/day and reduce to lowest daily or alternate-day dose that stabilizes symptoms	■ Bronchodilator as needed for symptoms (see step 1) up to 3 times a day
STEP 3 **Moderate** **Persistent**	■ Daily antiinflammatory medication. Either: – Medium-dose inhaled corticosteroid with spacer/holding chamber and face mask OR, once control is established: – Medium-dose inhaled corticosteroid and nedocromil OR: – Medium-dose inhaled corticosteroid and long-acting bronchodilator (theophylline)	■ Bronchodilator as needed for symptoms (see step 1) up to 3 times a day
STEP 2 **Mild** **Persistent**	■ Daily antiinflammatory medication. Either: – Cromolyn (nebulizer is preferred; or MDI) or nedocromil (MDI only) tid–qid – Infants and young children usually begin with a trial of cromolyn or nedocromil OR: – Low-dose inhaled corticosteroid with spacer/holding chamber and face mask	■ Bronchodilator as needed for symptoms (see step 1)

STEP 1
Mild
Intermittent
	■ No daily medicine needed.	■ Bronchodilator as needed for symptoms < 2 times a week. Intensity of treatment will depend upon severity of exacerbation. Either:
		
		– Inhaled short-acting beta$_2$-agonist by nebulizer or face mask and spacer/holding chamber
		OR:
		– Oral beta$_2$-agonist for symptoms
		
		■ With viral respiratory infection:
		
		– Bronchodilator q 4–6 hours up to 24 hours (longer with physician consult) but, in general, repeat no more than once every 6 weeks
		– Consider systemic corticosteroid
		  • If current exacerbation is severe
		  OR:
		  • If patient has history of previous severe exacerbations

Notes:

■ Gain control as quickly as possible: then decrease treatment to the least medication necessary to maintain control. Gaining control may be accomplished by either starting treatment at the step most appropriate to the initial severity of their condition or by starting at a higher level of therapy (eg, a course of systemic corticosteroids or higher dose of inhaled corticosteroids).

■ A rescue course of systemic corticosteroid (prednisolone) may be needed at any time and step.

■ In general, use of short-acting beta$_2$-agonist > 3 or 4 times in 1 day or regular use on a daily basis indicates the need for additional therapy.

■ It is important to remember that there are very few studies on asthma therapy for infants.

■ The stepwise approach presents guidelines to assist clinical decision making. Asthma is highly variable; clinicians should tailor specific medication plans to the needs and circumstances of individual patients.

■ Consultation with an asthma specialist is recommended for patients in this age group requiring step 3 or step 4 care. Consider consultation for patients in this age group requiring step 2 care.

↓ Step down

Review treatment every 1 to 6 months. If control is sustained for at least 3 months, a gradual stepwise reduction in treatment may be possible.

↑ Step up

If control is not achieved, consider step up. But first: review patient medication technique, adherence, and environmental control (avoidance of allergens or other precipitant factors).

Figure A254.

STEPWISE APPROACH FOR MANAGING ASTHMA IN ADULTS AND CHILDREN OVER 5 YEARS OLD

Goals of Asthma Treatment

- Prevent chronic and troublesome symptoms (eg, coughing or breathlessness in the night, in the early morning, or after exertion)

- Maintain (near) "normal" pulmonary function

- Maintain normal activity levels (including exercise and other physical activity)

- Prevent recurrent exacerbations of asthma and minimize the need for emergency department visits or hospitalizations

- Provide optimal pharmacotherapy with minimal or no adverse effects

- Meet patients' and families' expectation of and satisfaction with asthma care

Classification of Severity: Clinical Features Before Treatment[a]

	Symptoms[b]	Nighttime Symptoms	Lung Function
STEP 4 Severe Persistent	■ Continual symptoms ■ Limited physical activity ■ Frequent exacerbations	Frequent	■ FEV_1 or PEF $\leq$ 60% predicted ■ PEF variability > 30%
STEP 3 Moderate Persistent	■ Daily symptoms ■ Daily use of inhaled short-acting beta$_2$-agonist ■ Exacerbations affect activity ■ Exacerbations $\geq$ 2 times a week; may last days	> 1 time a week	■ FEV_1 or PEF > 60% $\leq$ 80% predicted ■ PEF variability > 30%
STEP 2 Mild Persistent	■ Symptoms > 2 times a week but < 1 time a day ■ Exacerbations may affect activity	> 2 times a month	■ FEV_1 or PEF $\geq$ 80% predicted ■ PEF variability 20–30%
STEP 1 Mild Intermittent	■ Symptoms $\leq$ 2 times a week ■ Asymptomatic and normal PEF between exacerbations ■ Exacerbations brief (from a few hours to a few days); intensity may vary	$\leq$ 2 times a month	■ FEV_1 or PEF $\geq$ 80% predicted ■ PEF variability < 20%

[a] The presence of one of the features of severity is sufficient to place a patient in that category. An individual should be assigned to the most severe grade in which any feature occurs. The characteristics noted in this figure are general and may overlap because asthma is highly variable. Furthermore, an individual's classification may change over time.

[b] Patients at any level of severity can have mild, moderate, or severe exacerbations. Some patients with intermittent asthma experience severe and life-threatening exacerbations separated by long periods of normal lung function and no symptoms.

Figure A254. *Continued.*

Preferred treatments are in bold print.

	Long-Term Control	Quick Relief	Education
STEP 4 **Severe** **Persistent**	Daily medications: ■ **Antiinflammatory: Inhaled corticosteroid (high dose)** and ■ Long-acting bronchodilator: either long-acting inhaled beta$_2$-agonist, sustained-release theophylline, or long-acting beta$_2$-agonist tablets AND ■ Corticosteroid tablets or syrup long term (2 mg/kg/day, generally do not exceed 60 mg/day).	■ Short-acting bronchodilator: **inhaled beta$_2$-agonists** as needed for symptoms. ■ Intensity of treatment will depend on severity of exacerbation; see "Managing Exacerbations of Asthma." ■ Use of short-acting inhaled beta$_2$-agonists on a daily basis, or increasing use, indicates the need for additional long-term-control therapy.	Steps 2 and 3 actions plus: ■ Refer to individual education/counseling

STEP 3
Moderate
Persistent
	Daily medication:
	
	■ Either
	
	  – **Antiinflammatory: inhaled corticosteroid (medium dose)** OR
	
	  – Inhaled corticosteroid (low-medium dose) and add a long-acting bronchodilator, especially for nighttime symptoms: either **long-acting Inhaled beta$_2$-agonist**, sustained-release theophylline, or long-acting beta$_2$-agonist tablets.
	
	■ If needed
	
	  – Antiinflammatory: inhaled corticosteroids (medium-high dose) AND
	
	  – Long-acting bronchodilator, especially for nighttime symptoms; either **long-acting Inhaled beta$_2$-agonist**, sustained-release theophylline, or long-acting beta$_2$-agonist tablets.
		■ Short-acting bronchodilator: **inhaled beta$_2$-agonists** as needed for symptoms.
		
		■ Intensity of treatment will depend on severity of exacerbation; see "Managing Exacerbations of Asthma."
		
		■ Use of short-acting inhaled beta$_2$-agonists on a daily basis, or increasing use, indicates the need for additional long-term-control therapy.
			Step 1 actions plus:
			
			■ Teach self-monitoring
			
			■ Refer to group education if available
			
			■ Review and update self-management plan

Figure A254. *Continued.*

STEPWISE APPROACH FOR MANAGING ASTHMA IN ADULTS AND CHILDREN OVER 5 YEARS OLD: TREATMENT (CONTINUED)

Preferred treatments are in bold print.

	Long-Term Control	Quick Relief	Education
STEP 2 **Mild** **Persistent**	Daily medication: ■ **Antiinflammatory: either inhaled corticosteroid** (low doses) or **cromolyn or nedocromil** (children usually begin with a trial of cromolyn or nedocromil). ■ Sustained-release theophylline to serum concentration of 5–15 μg/mL is an alternative. Zafirlukast or zileuton may also be considered for patients ≥ 12 years of age, although their position in therapy is not fully established.	■ Short-acting bronchodilator: **inhaled beta₂-agonists** as needed for symptoms. ■ Intensity of treatment will depend on severity of exacerbation; see "Managing Exacerbations of Asthma." ■ Use of short-acting inhaled beta₂-agonists on a daily basis, or increasing use, indicates the need for additional long-term-control therapy.	Step 1 actions plus: ■ Teach self-monitoring ■ Refer to group education if available ■ Review and update self-management plan
STEP 1 **Mild** **Intermittent**	■ No daily medication needed.	■ Short-acting bronchodilator: **inhaled beta₂-agonists** as needed for symptoms. ■ Intensity of treatment will depend on severity of exacerbation; see "Managing Exacerbations of Asthma." ■ Use of short-acting inhaled beta₂-agonists more than 2 times a week may indicate the need to initiate long-term-control therapy.	■ Teach basic facts about asthma ■ Teach inhaler/spacer/ holding chamber technique ■ Discuss roles of medications ■ Develop self-management plan ■ Develop action plan for when and how to take rescue actions ■ Discuss appropriate environmental control measures to avoid exposure to known allergens and irritants. (See component 4.)

Step down
↓ Review treatment every 1–6 months; a gradual stepwise reduction in treatment may be possible.

↑ Step up
If control is not maintained, consider step up. First, review patient medication technique, adherence, and environmental control (avoidance of allergens or other factors that contribute to asthma severity).

Notes:
■ The stepwise approach presents general guidelines to assist clinical decisionmaking; it is not intended to be a specific prescription. Asthma is highly variable; clinicians should tailor specific medication plans to the needs and circumstances of individual patients.
■ Gain control as quickly as possible; then decrease treatment to the least medication necessary to maintain control. Gaining control may be accomplished either by starting treatment at the step most appropriate to the initial severity of their condition or by starting at a higher level of therapy (eg, a course of systemic corticosteroids or higher dose of inhaled corticosteroids).
■ A rescue course of systemic corticosteroid may be needed at any time and at any step.
■ Some patients with intermittent asthma experience severe and life-threatening exacerbations separated by long periods of normal lung function and no symptoms. This may be especially common with exacerbations provoked by respiratory infections. A short course of systemic corticosteroids is recommended.
■ At each step, patients should control their environment to avoid or control factors that make their asthma worse (eg, allergens, irritants); this requires specific diagnosis and education.
■ Referral to an asthma specialist for consultation or comanagement is recommended if there are difficulties achieving or maintaining control of asthma or if the patient requires step 4 care. Referral may be considered if the patient requires step 3 care (see also component 1–Initial Assessment and Diagnosis).

Figure A254. Continued. Reprinted with permission from National Heart, Lung, and Blood Institute. Publication No. 97-4051A, May 1997. Bethesda, MD: National Institutes of Health.

TABLE A255-1. USUAL DOSAGES FOR QUICK-RELIEF MEDICATIONS

Medication	Dosage Form	Adult Dose	Child Dose	Comments
		Short-Acting Inhaled Beta₂-Agonists		
	MDIs			
Albuterol	■ 90 µg/puff, 200 puffs	■ 2 puffs 5 minutes prior to exercise	■ 1–2 puffs 5 minutes prior to exercise	■ An increasing use or lack of expected effect indicates diminished control of asthma.
Albuterol HFA	■ 90 µg/puff, 200 puffs	■ 2 puffs tid–qid	■ 2 puffs tid–qid	■ Not generally recommended for long-term treatment. Regular use on a daily basis indicates the need for additional long-term-control therapy.
Bitolterol	■ 370 µg/puff, 300 puffs			■ Differences in potency exist so that all products are essentially equipotent on a per puff basis.
Pirbuterol	■ 200 µg/puff, 400 puffs			■ May double usual dose for mild exacerbations.
Terbutaline	■ 200 µg/puff, 300 puffs			■ Nonselective agents (ie, epinephrine, isoproterenol, metaproterenol) are not recommended due to their potential for excessive cardiac stimulation, especially at high doses.
	DPIs			
Albuterol Rotahaler	■ 200 µg/capsule	■ 1–2 capsules q 4–6 hours as needed and prior to exercise	■ 1 capsule q 4–6 hours as needed and prior to exercise	
	Nebulizer solution			
Albuterol	■ 5 mg/mL (0.5%)	■ 1.25–5 mg (0.25–1 cc) in 2–3 cc of saline q 4–8 hours	■ 0.05 mg/kg (min 1.25 mg, max 2.5 mg) in 2–3 cc of saline q 4–6 hours	■ May mix with cromolyn or ipratropium nebulizer solutions. May double dose for mild exacerbations.
Bitolterol	■ 2 mg/mL (0.2%)	■ 0.5–3.5 mg (0.25–1 cc) in 2–3 cc of saline q 4–8 hours	■ Not established	■ May not mix with other nebulizer solutions.
		Anticholinergics		
	MDIs			
Ipratropium	■ 18 µg/puff, 200 puffs	■ 2–3 puffs q 6 hours	■ 1–2 puffs q 6 hours	■ Evidence is lacking for producing added benefit to beta₂-agonists in long-term asthma therapy.
	Nebulizer solution			
	■ 0.25 mg/mL (0.025%)	■ 0.25–0.5 mg q 6 hours	■ 0.25 mg q 6 hours	
		Systemic Corticosteroids		
Methylprednisolone	■ 2, 4, 8, 16, 32 mg tablets	■ Short course "burst": 40–60 mg/day as single of 2 divided doses for 3–10 days	■ Short course "burst": 1–2 mg/kg/day, maximum 60 mg/day, for 3–10 days	■ Short courses or "bursts" are effective for establishing control when initiating therapy or during a period of gradual deterioration.
Prednisolone	■ 5 mg tabs, 5 mg/5 cc, 15 mg/5 cc			■ The burst should be continued until patient achieves 80% PEF personal best or symptoms resolve. This usually requires 3–10 days but may require longer. There is no evidence that tapering the dose following improvement prevents relapse.
Prednisone	■ 1, 2.5, 5, 10, 20, 25 mg tabs; 5 mg/cc, 5 mg/5 cc			

TABLE A255-2. USUAL DOSAGES FOR LONG-TERM-CONTROL MEDICATIONS

Medication	Dosage Form	Adult Dose	Child Dose	Comments
		Systemic Corticosteroids		
Methylprednisolone	2, 4, 8, 16, 32 mg tablets	7.5–60 mg daily in a single dose or qod as needed for control	0.25–2 mg/kg daily in single dose or qod as needed for control	For long-term treatment of severe persistent asthma, administer single dose in A.M. either daily or on alternate days (alternate-day therapy may produce less adrenal suppression). If daily doses are required, one study suggests improved efficacy and no increase in adrenal suppression when administered at 3:00 P.M.
Prednisolone	5 mg tabs, 5 mg/5 cc, 15 mg/5 cc	Short-course "burst": 40–60 mg per day as single or 2 divided doses for 3–10 days	Short course "burst": 1–2 mg/kg/day, maxmum 60 mg/day, for 3–10 days	Short courses or "bursts" are effective for establishing control when initiating therapy or during a period of gradual deterioration.
Prednisone	1, 2.5, 5, 10, 20, 25 mg tabs; 5 mg/cc, 5 mg/5 cc			The burst should be continued until patient achieves 80% PEF personal best or symptoms resolve. This usually requires 3–10 days but may require longer. There is no evidence that tapering the dose following improvement prevents relapse.
		Cromolyn and Nedocromil		
Cromolyn	MDI 1 mg/puff Nebulizer solution 20 mg/ampule	2–4 puffs tid–qid 1 ampule tid–qid	1–2 puffs tid–qid 1 ampule tid–qid	One dose prior to exercise or allergen exposure provides effective prophylaxis for 1–2 hours.
Nedocromil	MDI 1.75 mg/puff	2–4 puffs bid–qid	1–2 puffs bid–qid	See cromolyn above.
		Long-Acting Beta₂-Agonists		
Salmeterol	*Inhaled* MDI 21 µg/puff, 60 or 120 puffs	2 puffs q 12 hours	1–2 puffs q 12 hours	May use one dose nightly for symptoms.
	DPI 50 µg/blister	1 blister q 12 hours	1 blister q 12 hours	Should not be used as a rescue inhaler for symptom relief or for exacerbations.
- Sustained-release albuterol	*Tablet* 4 mg tablet	4 mg q 12 hours	0.3–0.6 mg/kg/day, not to exceed 8 mg/day	
		Methylxanthines		
Theophylline (numerous manufacturers)	Liquids Sustained-release tablets and capsules	Starting dose 10 mg/kg/day up to 300 mg max; usual max 800 mg/day	Starting dose 10 mg/kg/day; usual max: ≥ 1 year of age: 16 mg/kg/day	Adjust dosage to achieve serum concentration of 5–15 µg/mL at steady-state (at least 48 hours on same dosage).

(continued)

TABLE A255-2. *(Continued)*

Medication	Dosage Form	Adult Dose	Child Dose	Comments
		Methylxanthines	<1 year: 0.2 (age in weeks) + 5 = mg/kg/day	Due to wide interpatient variability in the theophylline metabolic clearance, routine serum theophylline level monitoring is important. See below for factors that can affect levels.

FACTORS AFFECTING SERUM THEOPHYLLINE CONCENTRATIONS

Factor	Decreases Theophylline Concentrations	Increases Theophylline Concentrations	Recommended Action
Food	↓ or delays absorption of some sustained-release theophylline (SRT) products	↑ rate of absorption (fatty foods) products	Select theophylline preparation that is not affected by food.
Diet	↑ metabolism (high protein)	↓ metabolism (high carbohydrate)	Inform patients that major changes in diet are not recommended while taking theophylline.
Systemic, febrile viral illness (eg, influenza)		↓ metabolism	Decrease theophylline dose according to serum concentration level. Decrease dose by 50% if serum concentration measurement is not available.
Hypoxia, cor pulmonale, and decompensated congestive heart failure, cirrhosis		↓ metabolism	Decrease dose according to serum concentration level.
Age	↑ metabolism (1–9 years)	↓ metabolism (< 6 months, elderly)	Adjust dose according to serum concentration level.
Phenobarbital, phenytoin, carbamazepine	↑ metabolism		Increase dose according to serum concentration level.
Cimetidine		↓ metabolism	Use alternative H_2 blocker (eg, famotidine or ranitidine).
Macrolides: TAO, erythromycin, clarithromycin		↓ metabolism	Use alternative antibiotic or adjust theophylline dose.
Quinolones: ciprofloxacin, enoxacin, pefloxacin		↓ metabolism	Use alternative antibiotic or adjust theophylline dose. Circumvent with ofloxacin if quinolone therapy is required.
Rifampin	↑ metabolism		Increase dose according to serum concentration level.
Ticlopidine		↓ metabolism	Decrease dose according to serum concentration level.
Smoking	↑ metabolism		Advise patient to stop smoking; increase dose according to serum concentration level.

Reprinted with permission from National Heart, Lung, and Blood Institute. Publication No. 97-4051A, May 1997. Bethesda, MD: National Institutes of Health.

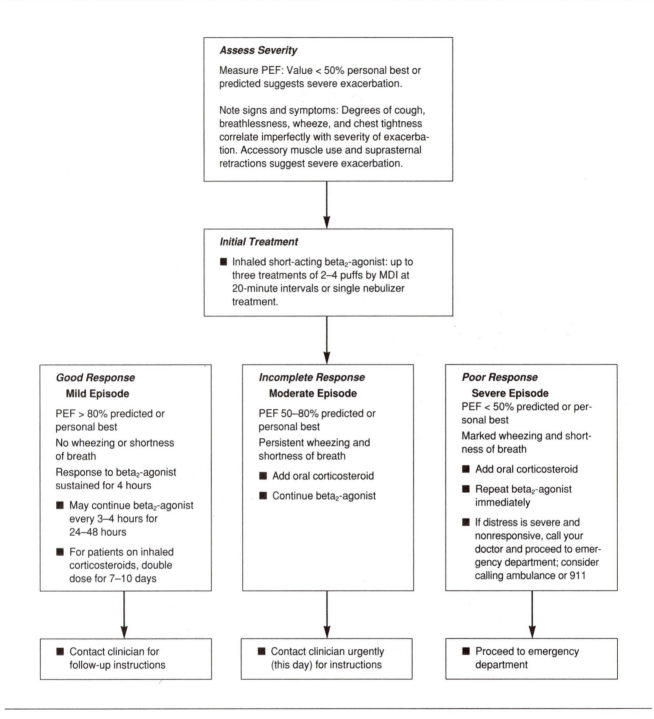

Figure A257. Management of Asthma Exacerbations: Home Treatment. *(Reprinted with permission from National Heart, Lung, and Blood Institute. Publication No. 97-4051A, May 1997. Bethesda, MD: National Institutes of Health.)*

Neurologic

CASES AND QUESTIONS

Questions 284–288

Tom is a 15-year-old who developed a headache at school today. This headache is located bilaterally over his temporal area. He denies photophobia and there has been no vomiting. He was entirely well prior to this afternoon. He has no previous history of headaches.

284. The most critical portion of the evaluation of headaches in children and adolescents is

   (A) A complete examination of cranial nerves
   (B) A complete headache history
   (C) A complete physical examination
   (D) Neuroimaging

285. Other questions in this adolescent's history that would be important to ask concerning his headache include

   (A) Family history of headaches
   (B) Alcohol, illicit drug, and medication use
   (C) History of headache when arising from sleep
   (D) All of the above

Tom describes the pain as "a dull ache." He admits to a heavy after-school sports and activity schedule. He is currently involved in a major role in a school drama performance. His entire physical examination including his neurologic examination is benign except for a dull, aching bifrontal headache and muscle tightness in his shoulders. He is nontoxic appearing and afebrile, and his blood pressure is 100/72.

286. Which type of headache is Tom most likely experiencing?

   (A) Muscle contraction headache
   (B) Vascular headache
   (C) Traction or inflammatory headache
   (D) Mixed headache

287. Effective management of headache in this adolescent patient would include

   (A) Appropriate medication or other intervention
   (B) Explanation of the cause and expected course of the headache
   (C) Elimination of headache triggers
   (D) All of the above

288. Headaches are unusual and more indicative of serious underlying disease in

   (A) Adolescents
   (B) Children of all ages
   (C) Preschool-age children
   (D) School-age children

Questions 289–291

Abigail is a 20-month-old female whose dad has brought her to the clinic today following a fall, which occurred approximately 1 hour ago. The child was climbing up onto a plastic toddler climbing structure at home when she fell and hit her head.

289. Other questions in the history that would be important to ask concerning this child's injury include

(A) The mechanism of injury
(B) Immunization status
(C) Previous injury history related to falls
(D) Gross motor achievements to date

The fall was from less than 2 feet. The father witnessed her land on the back of her head. She cried vigorously and immediately after the fall. She vomited once after crying. Abigail's physical and neurologic examinations are all intact. She has been interactive and playful in the clinic with a normal gait and normal coordination exam.

290. All the following are consistent with a mild head injury EXCEPT

(A) No loss of consciousness
(B) Persistent vomiting after injury
(C) Absence of neurologic deficit
(D) Mild headache

291. Appropriate management of this child's mild head injury would include

(A) Transfer to a hospital for immediate emergency care
(B) Skull x-rays followed by 1–2 hours of observation at the clinic
(C) Careful at-home observation by parents with head injury precautions
(D) None of the above

Questions 292–294

Philip, 9 years old, has an unusual recurring behavior. His parents noted that he began to lick his lips several times a day accompanied by shrugging of his shoulders. In addition, he will make sniffling noises, blink his eyes, chew on his shirt with his teeth, and rub his chin on his chest. This behavior began suddenly and has occurred over a 3–4 month period. His schoolwork has not deteriorated. The parents report he has always had trouble paying attention in class and has trouble completing tasks. His PE, including a neuromuscular examination, is entirely normal although he licks his lips frequently during the exam.

292. Which of the following statements regarding tic disorders is *false?*

(A) Commonly presents between ages 6 and 12 years
(B) More common in females than in males
(C) History is often familial
(D) Cause is unknown

293. Gilles de la Tourette's syndrome is characterized by

1. Simple transient tics
2. Multiple motor and vocal tics displayed over time
3. Chronic tics

(A) 1 only
(B) 2 only
(C) 3 only
(D) 2 and 3 only

294. Which of the following psychobehavioral problems may be associated with Tourette's syndrome?

1. ADHD
2. Hallucinations
3. Obsessive–compulsive disorder
4. All of the above

(A) 2 only
(B) 3 only
(C) 1 and 3
(D) All of the above

Questions 295–299

Denise, an 18-month-old child, is seen today by the PNP following a visit last evening to a local emergency ward (EW). Denise was entirely well and active yesterday until dinnertime, when she became lethargic and her mother noted her to "be very hot." At that time Denise's temperature was 37.9°C (103.8°F) rectally. The parent left the room just to get Denise some acetaminophen. When she returned, she found Denise lying on her bed unresponsive and her body stiff. Denise's face and body then began to jerk intermittently. The parent immediately called 911; when EMTs arrived, the child was alert and responsive and the movements had ceased. She was taken to a local EW for evaluation and treatment. A septic workup and neurologic examination were normal. She was treated with amoxicillin for a left acute otitis media. She was discharged home with close follow-up.

295. Which of the following is *not* typical of a simple febrile seizure?

(A) Positive family history
(B) Seizure lasting more than 15 minutes
(C) Age of onset between 3 months and 5 years
(D) Most likely to occur with a rapid rise in body temperature

296. Which of the following seizure types carries the worst prognosis for future mental development?

(A) Absence seizures (petit mal)
(B) Febrile
(C) Generalized tonic–clonic seizure (grand mal)
(D) Infantile spasms

297. Appropriate management for this child would include all of the following EXCEPT

(A) Instruct parents on the treatment plan for fever.
(B) Advise parents to call if seizure recurs.
(C) Inform parents as to the overall risk of recurrence.
(D) Begin prophylactic anticonvulsant drug therapy.

298. The appropriate dose of acetaminophen for this child would be

(A) 1 mg/kg per dose up to five doses in 24 hours
(B) 5 mg/kg per dose up to five doses in 24 hours
(C) 15 mg/kg per dose up to five doses in 24 hours
(D) None of the above

299. The appropriate dose of ibuprofen for this child if her temperature was below 39.3°C (102.5°F) would be

(A) 1 mg/kg/dose every 8 hours
(B) 10 mg/kg/dose every 8 hours
(C) 15 mg/kg/dose every 8 hours
(D) None of the above

ANSWERS AND RATIONALES

284. **(B)** A thorough headache history is essential since the diagnosis depends almost entirely on the history. Since the majority of patients with headache will have an entirely normal physical and neurologic examination, the history becomes the primary part of the evaluation (Dunn & Purvin, 1990; Weiss, 1993).

285. **(D)** Essential components of the headache history include assessment of the following: duration, frequency, possible triggers, location, quality of pain, severity, associated symptoms, history of head trauma, family history, any psychological symptoms, progression of headache over time, home management, and alcohol, illicit drug, and medication use.

286. **(A)** The most common headache with onset in adolescence is tension headache. Unlike the vascular headache of migraine, the typical tension headache is frontal with no associated symptoms and no prodrome. It is diffuse, mild to moderate in intensity and is chronic in nature. Physical and neurologic examination in tension headache is normal. (See Table A286.)

287. **(D)** Treatment of headaches in the adolescent patient is individualized. Headache management for this adolescent would include identification and elimination of headache triggers, evaluation of the headaches over time including use of a headache diary, explanation of the cause and course of the headache, and medications (Dunn & Purvin, 1990).

288. **(C)** Headache is not a usual symptom or complaint in very young children. Headache in a child age 3–10 years—the peak age for brain tumors—is unusual and may be indicative of serious underlying disease.

289. **(A)** The most important step in evaluating a child with head injury is to take an accurate and detailed history from either the child or a reliable witness to the accident. Information such as how the child fell and from what distance is critical in determining the severity of the head injury.

TABLE A286. FEATURES OF COMMON HEADACHES IN CHILDHOOD

Muscle contraction/tension
  Chronic and protracted
  Diffuse squeezing or pressure sensation
  Band distribution around head
  No prodrome
  Associated anxiety and depression
  Environmental triggers prominent

Migraine
  Acute, paroxysmal
  Unilateral or bilateral
  Temporal, retro-orbital, or frontal
  Throbbing or pulsating quality
  May have prodrome
  Positive family history (75%)
  Environmental triggers occasionally

Increased intracranial pressure/traction headache
  Intermittent or chronic
  Progressively increasing severity or frequency through time
  Positional pain
  Diffuse pressure
  No prodrome
  Associated focal or lateralized neurologic deficits

Reprinted with permission from Seay, A.R., & Janas, J. (1997). Neurologic and muscular disorders. In G.B. Merenstein, D.W. Kaplan, & A.A. Rosenberg, eds. Handbook of pediatrics (18th ed., p. 655). Stamford, CT: Appleton & Lange.

290. **(B)** Mild to moderate head injuries are far more common than severe injuries in pediatrics. Infants and children can be assessed with a thorough history and physical examination with emphasis on vital signs, head and neck, and neurologic exams. The Glasgow Coma Scale (GCS) is a convenient way to evaluate a child's level of consciousness and monitor neurologic signs (Table A290). In cases of mild head injury (no loss of consciousness, a GCS of 15, no focal neurologic deficits, and no palpable depressed skull fracture), it is not uncommon to see a child who has vomited once or even twice. The infant or child that has persistent vomiting or starts vomiting again several hours after the accident would warrant a neurosurgical evaluation and CT scan (Goldstein & Powers, 1994; Schutzman, 1996).

291. **(C)** The child with minor head injury, who is alert with no other injuries, has a normal neurologic examination, and a reliable caregiver to monitor and return the patient should complication arise, can be managed at home. Parents or caregivers should be given instructions (preferably written) that include specific indications for contacting the health care provider or taking the child to the emergency room.

292. **(B)** Many cases of of Gilles de la Tourette's syndrome are familial, and the prevalence of tics is higher in males than in females. The onset commonly presents between ages 6 and 12 years. The cause remains unknown, although tics are thought to be related to an abnormality within the deep structures of the cerebral hemispheres.

293. **(D)** Tourette's is a common cause of tics in childhood. It is characterized by multiple motor and vocal tics over time that are present for longer than 1 year. The onset of tics is before 21 years of age and not associated with other known conditions.

294. **(C)** Other psychobehavioral problems, such as attention deficit hyperactivity disorder (ADHD) and obsessive–compulsive behav-

TABLE A290. PEDIATRIC MODIFICATION OF GLASGOW COMA SCALE (GCS) BY AGE OF PATIENT[a]

Glasgow Coma Score	Pediatric Modification	
Eye Opening **≥1 year**	**0–1 year**	
4 Spontaneously	4 Spontaneously	
3 To verbal command	3 To shout	
2 To pain	2 To pain	
1 No response	1 No response	
Best Motor Response **≥1 year**	**0–1 year**	
6 Obeys		
5 Localizes pain	5 Localizes pain	
4 Flexion withdrawal	4 Flexion withdrawal	
3 Flexion abnormal (decorticate)	3 Flexion abnormal (decorticate)	
2 Extension (decerebrate)	2 Extension (decerebrate)	
1 No response	1 No response	
Best Verbal Response **>5 years**	**0–2 years**	**2–5 years**
5 Oriented and converses	5 Cries appropriately, smiles, coos	5 Appropriate words and phrases
4 Disoriented and converses	4 Cries	4 Inappropriate words
3 Inappropriate words	3 Inappropriate crying/screaming	3 Cries/screams
2 Incomprehensible sounds	2 Grunts	2 Grunts
1 No response	1 No response	1 No response

[a] Score is the sum of the individual scores from eye opening, best verbal response, and best motor response, using age-specific criteria. GCS of 13–15 indicates mild head injury, GCS of 9–12 indicates moderate head injury, and GCS < 8 indicates severe head injury.
Reprinted with permission from Barkin, R.M., & Rosen, P. (1994). Emergency pediatrics: A guide to ambulatory care (4th ed.). St. Louis: Mosby.

iors, may be associated with Tourette's syndrome. However, not all affected children have these associated problems.

295.   **(B)** Criteria for febrile seizures include (1) noncentral nervous systems infection, (2) fever of 102°F (38°C), and (3) age 3 months to 5 years of age. Greater than 90% of febrile seizures are generalized and less than 5 minutes in length. Early otitis media, pharyngitis, adenitis, and roseola are classic causes of febrile seizures. Febrile seizures occur in 2–3% of children.

296.   **(D)** The peak age of onset of infantile spasms is 3–8 months of age and 86% of infants will experience the onset of seizures before age 1 year of age. Infantile spasms are characterized by a brief contraction of the trunk, neck, and arm muscles, followed by sustained muscle contractions. Mental retardation may accompany or follow the onset of infantile spasms (Painter & Bergman, 1994). (See Table A296.)

297.   **(D)** Continuous prophylactic anticonvulsant therapy following a first febrile seizure is not generally recommended; however, long-term prophylaxis may be considered in children with multiple risk factors for future seizures (Rosenstein & Fosarelli, 1997). Parents should be educated and instructed in fever reduction and control.

298.   **(C)** The appropriate dosage of acetaminophen in infants and children is 10–15 mg/kg/dose every 4–6 hours as needed, not to exceed 5 doses in 24 hours (Taketomo, Hodding, & Kraus, 1996).

299.   **(D)** The appropriate dosage of ibuprofen in children 6 months to 12 years of age for temperature < 102.5°F (39°C) is 5 mg/kg/dose; give every 6–8 hours as needed. For temperatures > 102.5°F (39°C) the correct dosage is 10 mg/kg/dose; give every 6–8 hours as needed (Taketomo, Hodding, & Kraus, 1996).

TABLE A296. COMMON SEIZURE TYPES IN CHILDREN

Seizure Type	Age at Onset	Clinical Manifestations	Treatment
Partial			
Simple partial (focal motor, sensory, autonomic)	Any age	No disturbance of consciousness. May involve any part of the body. May spread in fixed pattern (Jacksonian) and become generalized.	Carbamazepine, phenytoin, phenobarbital or primidone; valproic acid may be a useful adjunct.
Complex partial	Any age	Associated with impairment of consciousness. The aura may be sensation of fear, epigastric discomfort, odd smell or taste, visual or auditory hallucination. Proceeds to period of altered behavior which may be characterized by walking in a daze, facial movements such as eye blinking, lip smacking, chewing or other automatisms. If the seizure consists solely of an aura, it is classified as a partial seizure. Complex partial seizures may also generalize.	Carbamazepine, phenytoin, phenobarbital or primidone. Valproic acid may be a useful adjunct.
Generalized			
Tonic–clonic	Any age	Loss of consciousness, ± bladder/bowel incontinence, postictal confusion.	Phenobarbital, carbamazepine, phenytoin, valproic acid, primidone.
Absence	3–15 years	Lapses of consciousness lasting about 10 seconds. Often in clusters. May see automatisms of face and hands.	Ethosuximide or valproic acid.
Myoclonic	Any age (usually 2–7 years)	Abrupt contractions of one or more muscle groups, singly or irregularly repetitive. Usually no or only brief loss of consciousness.	Valproic acid, clonazepam, ethosuximide. Imipramine is adjunct. Diazepam. Ketogenic or medium chain triglyceride diet. ACTH or corticosteroids in West's syndrome.

Reprinted with permission from Seay, A.R., & Janas, J. (1997). Neurologic and muscular disorders. In G.B. Merenstein, D.W. Kaplan, & A.A. Rosenberg, eds. Handbook of pediatrics (18th ed., p. 633). Stamford, CT: Appleton & Lange.

Gastrointestinal

CASES AND QUESTIONS

Questions 300–304

Thirty-month-old Tamra is brought in by her parents for a complaint of diarrhea for the past 4 weeks. The stools are reported to occur between three and six times a day, are light in color, and are foul-smelling. The diarrhea was preceded by an episode of acute gastroenteritis. The child is otherwise healthy and has had normal growth, good appetite, and no reports of discomfort except for straining while stooling. The physical exam is noncontributory and negative for abdominal tenderness, distention, and palpable stool.

300. Which of the following laboratory tests would be *most* helpful in determining the cause of this child's diarrhea?

    (A) Stool culture
    (B) Stool exam for ova and parasite
    (C) Stool pH
    (D) All of the above

301. Other elements of the history that would be *most* helpful in determining the cause of this child's diarrhea would be

    (A) Recent immunizations
    (B) Family history of cystic fibrosis
    (C) Detailed dietary history
    (D) Present developmental milestones

302. A common cause of chronic diarrhea in otherwise healthy toddlers in the United States is

    (A) Celiac disease
    (B) Inflammatory bowel disease (IBD)

    (C) Bacterial gastroenteritis (GE)
    (D) Chronic nonspecific diarrhea (CNSD)

303. An important risk factor in evaluating a child for inflammatory bowel disease (IBD) is

    (A) A family history of IBD
    (B) A family history of atopic disease
    (C) Recent salmonella infection
    (D) Evidence of iron deficiency anemia

304. A common presenting symptom of inflammatory bowel disease (IBD) in children is

    (A) Joint inflammation
    (B) Growth failure
    (C) Unexplained fever
    (D) Renal calculi

Questions 305–309

One-year-old Molly is sent home from day care with fever and vomiting. She presents on the second day of illness with a history of watery diarrhea, temperature of 38.3°C (101.0°F), loss of appetite, and two episodes of vomiting. She has been taking sips of apple juice. The history reveals that two other children at day care were out recently with similar illnesses. On exam she weighs 10 kg, her mucous membranes are dry, her skin turgor is normal, she is alert but irritable, and her abdomen is soft with active bowel sounds.

305. Molly's diarrheal illness is most likely due to which of these frequently occurring enteric pathogens?

    (A) *Shigella*
    (B) *Campylobacter jejuni*
    (C) *Escherichia coli*
    (D) *Rotavirus*

306. Shigellosis can cause significant complications. All of the following complications are known to occur EXCEPT

    (A) Dehydration
    (B) Neurotoxicity
    (C) Hepatitis
    (D) Bacteremia

307. The approximate fluid deficit in this moderately dehydrated infant is:

    (A) 200–400 mL
    (B) 400–600 mL
    (C) 600–800 mL
    (D) 800–1000 mL

308. What is the most common parasitic gastroenteritis in the United States?

    (A) *Clostridium difficile*
    (B) *Giardia lamblia*
    (C) *Escherichia coli*
    (D) None of the above

309. Which of the following therapeutics would be most appropriate for children with an acute diarrheal illness?

    (A) Half-strength formula
    (B) Discontinuation of solid foods until stool is formed
    (C) Bismuth subsalicylate
    (D) Continue breast-feeding

Questions 310–314

An 18-year-old college freshman presents to college health with an 8-hour history of abdominal pain that began in the periumbilical area and then localized to the right lower quadrant. She has been anorexic and nauseous and has had some diarrhea. She is sexually active and has been on oral contraceptive pills for the past 6 months. She denies a history of urinary tract infection, pregnancy, sexually transmitted diseases, or chronic illnesses. On physical exam, she has guarding of the right lower quadrant with generalized tenderness and no masses. Her temperature is 37.6°C (99.6°F) and her other vitals are normal.

310. Based on the history and physical exam, which of the following is the *most likely* diagnosis to consider?

    (A) Mittelschmertz
    (B) Ectopic pregnancy
    (C) Appendicitis
    (D) Gastroenteritis

311. Which of the following is *least* helpful in the evaluation of abdominal pain in children?

    (A) Urinalysis
    (B) Complete blood count
    (C) Temperature measurement
    (D) Pregnancy test

312. Of the following, the finding *most* suggestive of acute appendicitis is

    (A) Leukocytosis
    (B) Hematemesis
    (C) Positive psoas sign
    (D) Vomiting before the onset of pain

313. Acute abdominal pain with vaginal bleeding in a postmenarcheal patient would be *most* suggestive of which disorder?

    (A) Ectopic pregnancy
    (B) Appendicitis
    (C) Meckel's diverticulum
    (D) None of the above

314. Which of the following diagnostic tools would be most helpful in distinguishing the cause of acute testicular pain in boys?

    (A) Doppler exam of the scrotum
    (B) Complete blood count
    (C) Urinalysis
    (D) Radiograph of the pelvis

Questions 315–320

Seven-year-old Matt is referred by the school nurse for abdominal pain. He has repeatedly seen the school nurse over the course of 4 months complaining of stomachaches. He is in otherwise good health and has had no recent weight loss, fever, joint pain, rash, rectal bleeding, or recent known stress. He reports that his episodes occur daily, last between ½ and 3 hours, and are periumbilical in location. He also reports the pain occurs at different times of the day.

315. You suspect that this patient has recurrent abdominal pain (RAP). Which of the following findings supports this assessment?

    (A) Short duration of symptoms
    (B) Pain that frequently awakens the child at night
    (C) Fatigue
    (D) None of the above

316. A *true* statement regarding RAP is

    (A) Obesity is a risk factor.
    (B) Pain is frequently not related to activity or meals.
    (C) Guaiac-positive stools are commonly found.
    (D) The entity is commonly associated with depression.

317. Initial evaluation of this child to rule out organic disease requires which of the following tests?

    (A) A breath hydrogen test, CBC, ESR, guaiac stool
    (B) Abdominal radiograph, stool for ova and parasite, CBC
    (C) CBC, ESR, urinalysis, urine culture, guaiac stool
    (D) Throat culture, CBC, liver function tests

318. An overall goal of treatment of children with RAP is

    (A) To manage pain with nonsteroidal anti-inflammatory drugs (NSAIDs)
    (B) The restriction of normal activities
    (C) To improve intestinal motor activity
    (D) To encourage independence in dealing with the pain

319. Left lower quadrant pain in a child with RAP is most likely due to

    (A) Appendicitis
    (B) Cholelithiasis
    (C) Constipation
    (D) Peptic ulcer disease

320. Of the following, what is a common presentation of Hirschsprung's disease (congenital aganglionic megacolon) in infants?

    (A) Constipation
    (B) Guaiac-positive stools
    (C) Rectal prolapse
    (D) Imperforate anus

Questions 321–325

Jamie is a 5½-year-old boy who is brought by his mother for evaluation of 2 weeks of intermittent abdominal pain. A more detailed history reveals that the abdominal pain has actually been occurring for many months, but has recently gotten worse, prompting this visit. The child has difficulty describing the pain aside from locating it in his lower abdomen and commonly associating the pain to the postprandial period. He has not been awakened by the pain at night and has had no nausea or vomiting associated with it. He has had no recent febrile episodes, respiratory symptoms, rashes, or joint complaints. His mother believes he had been eating normally although with mildly decreased appetite in the past 2 weeks.

Upon more careful questioning, it is revealed that since starting kindergarten 6 weeks ago, Jamie has been acting in a somewhat sullen manner. The mother notices that when the pain is present, he will go off by himself. She reluctantly mentions that she has noticed frequent episodes of soiling in his underpants, which have occurred almost daily over the past 2 weeks. A surprise to his mother, Jamie reveals that he has only been having bowel movements every 3–5 days.

In reviewing Jamie's past history, it becomes evident that he had episodes of constipation in infancy and toddlerhood and was difficult to toilet-train. His mother states that he "almost seemed to hold back" in producing a stool. He eventually was toilet-trained at 3 years, 10 months. The rest of his review of systems and past medical history was noncontributory.

Jamie's physical exam was unremarkable except for a feeling of fullness in the left lower quadrant during the abdominal exam and a rectal exam that revealed firm pieces of stool in the rectal ampulla.

321. The definition of encopresis includes all of the following EXCEPT

  (A) Age greater than 4 years
  (B) Duration of symptoms for at least 1 month
  (C) More common in girls than boys
  (D) Involuntary defecation in unacceptable locations, especially in clothing

322. The most important factor in establishing a diagnosis of encopresis is:

  (A) Careful and detailed history
  (B) Careful and detailed physical exam
  (C) Examination of the child's stool
  (D) A barium enema

323. Common pathologic and psychological factors present in encopresis include all the following EXCEPT

  (A) Rectal hyposensitivity
  (B) A structural abnormality in the bowel
  (C) Behavior issues such as poor attention span or oppositional behavior
  (D) Fecal retention

324. Common therapeutic approaches that are appropriate in the treatment of encopresis include all the following EXCEPT

  (A) Stool softeners and bowel stimulants
  (B) Routine scheduling of toilet time
  (C) Aversive behavioral therapy
  (D) A behavioral reward system

325. The following statements regarding the prognosis and follow-up of encopresis are true EXCEPT

  (A) Frequent and careful follow-up are important to long-term success.
  (B) Within 6 months of starting treatment, most children with encopresis have a complete and long-lasting remission or are significantly improved.
  (C) Children who fail to respond to routine treatment may need more aggressive therapy including biofeedback or psychotherapy.
  (D) Recurrences during adolescence are common.

ANSWERS AND RATIONALES

300. **(D)** Children with chronic diarrhea should be evaluated through a stool culture for possible bacterial illness caused by *Campylobacter jejuni*. Other possible causes of diarrhea might include *Giardia lamblia*, which can be identified through a stool exam for ova and parasite. A test of the stool pH with nitrazine paper may suggest carbohydrate intolerance if the pH is less than 5.5 (Oski & Johnson, 1997).

301. **(C)** A detailed diet history is important in a child with chronic diarrhea, giving special attention to fiber, fluid, fat, and fruit juice intake. In response to the chronicity of the symptoms, parents will often restrict foods, thereby restricting fiber and other residue, while increasing the use of apple juice, which in fact has been found to promote diarrhea (Kneepkens & Hoekstra, 1996). Cystic fibrosis is unlikely in a child who has had otherwise normal growth and well-being. Recent immunizations have no bearing on this child's illness.

302. **(D)** Chronic nonspecific diarrhea (CNSD) is a condition that affects children between 1 and 5 years with symptoms of more than 3–4 weeks duration. The etiology is unknown, but the child is otherwise healthy with normal growth and no pain. The illness is frequently initiated by acute gastroenteritis or by an acute infection, which was treated by a broad-spectrum antibiotic that alters bacterial flora in the colon (Oski & Johnson, 1997; Kneepkens & Hoekstra, 1996). Cystic fibrosis and bacterial gastroenteritis, as well as malabsorption syndromes such as celiac disease, often interfere with a child's growth and overall well-being.

303. **(A)** A positive family history of inflammatory bowel disease (IBD) is the most consistent risk factor for children (Kirschner, 1996; Winesett, 1997). The remaining choices are not known to be risk factors for developing IBD in children.

304. **(B)** Ulcerative colitis (UC) is a chronic, relapsing, inflammatory disease of the colon and rectum. Growth failure is a common presenting symptom of the disease in children, although stools mixed with blood and mucus, along with lower abdominal cramping, may also be a presenting feature of the disease. Extra-intestinal manifestations, such as erythema nodosum, joint inflammation, and renal calculi, can occur in 25–35% of patients with UC (Winesett, 1997).

305. **(D)** Acute diarrheal illness caused by rotavirus is responsible for 25% of all cases in the United States. Peak incidence is in children 3–15 months of age during the winter months (Buzby, 1997). Vomiting is a common first symptom, with low-grade fever and profuse, watery diarrhea. Although other pathogens can cause acute diarrheal illness in children, they are not associated with a peak incidence in winter months.

306. **(C)** Shigellosis is the most common cause of bacterial diarrhea in children and occurs most often in the summer and fall months. The peak incidence of the illness is in children 1–4 years of age. Shigellosis is potentially a serious disease, particularly among children less than

2 years of age. It can cause dehydration, neurotoxicity with seizures, and bacteremia as major complications (Pickering, 1996).

307. **(D)** Oral rehydration therapy (ORT) is critical to the management of acute diarrheal illness. The American Academy of Pediatrics (AAP, 1996) recommends that oral rehydration solution contain 75–90 mEq/L sodium, 20–25 g/L glucose, and 20–30 mEq/L potassium. The amount of replacement therapy is dependent on the degree of dehydration. Infants with mild dehydration require 50 mL/kg of ORT, and those with moderate dehydration require 100 mL/kg. Therefore, this infant, weighing 10 kg, requires 100 mL × 10 kg = 1000 mL of fluids given over 4–6 hours (Buzby, 1997; AAP, 1996; Cohen, 1996).

308. **(B)** *Giardia lamblia* is the most common parasitic gastroenteritis in the United States. Transmission is by the fecal–oral route, although water supplies can also be a source of contamination. Children in day-care settings are at risk where outbreaks are common. Microscopic examination of fresh stool samples for ova and parasites will confirm diagnosis. *Campylobacter* is a bacterial cause of diarrheal illness in children and *Clostridium difficile* is a toxin-producing organism that causes diarrhea in children with altered bowel flora (Lieberman, 1994).

309. **(D)** In addition to oral rehydration therapy (ORT), recommendations for children with acute diarrhea include continuing breast-feeding and an age-appropriate diet that includes full-strength formula. Antidiarrheal agents such as bismuth subsalicylate (Pepto-Bismol) may have some palliative properties, but are generally not deemed necessary in the management of diarrheal illness in children (Galen, 1997).

310. **(C)** Acute appendicitis is the most common cause of emergency surgery in children. The progression of appendicitis to perforation is 10% by 24 hours and 50% by 48 hours, thereby making it important to diagnose and treat the patient early in the illness. The diagnosis of

appendicitis may be difficult to make in the adolescent female, but should be suspected with the classic signs and symptoms of right lower quadrant tenderness with guarding, accompanied by signs of peritoneal irritation (Oski & Johnson, 1997).

311. **(C)** Suggested laboratory studies of the patient with acute abdominal pain include a complete blood count (CBC), urinalysis, and pregnancy test in postmenarcheal patients. The abdominal radiograph may be helpful to evaluate the abdomen for bowel obstruction, calcification, ischemia, or free air. Ultrasound may also be useful to evaluate the patient for abdominal masses or to rule out gynecologic pathology (Stevenson & Ziegler, 1993).

312. **(C)** Appendicitis is characterized by varied symptomatology, depending on the age of the patient, the point in time he or she is evaluated during the course of the illness, and the location of the appendix in the abdomen. The classic signs and symptoms before perforation include right lower quadrant pain, low-grade fever, diarrhea, loss of appetite, vomiting, and decreased bowel sounds. Leukocytosis, a nonspecific finding, may occur due to the inflammatory process. A positive psoas sign, elicited by pain with extension of the hip to stretch the psoas muscle, is highly suggestive of appendicitis (Oski & Johnson, 1997; Stevenson & Ziegler, 1993).

313. **(A)** Ectopic pregnancy, although rare in the pediatric age group, should be considered in any postmenarcheal, sexually active client. The classic symptoms of abdominal pain, vaginal bleeding, and amenorrhea should raise suspicion, as well as a history of previous ectopic pregnancy, pelvic inflammatory disease, intrauterine device (IUD), previous abortion, tubal ligation, or infertility (Stevenson & Ziegler, 1993).

314. **(A)** Testicular torsion is a pediatric urologic emergency that requires prompt evaluation and referral. Any male patient who presents with acute lower abdominal pain should have his scrotum evaluated for evidence of torsion

(Stevenson & Ziegler, 1993). Testicular torsion can present at any age, but is more common at or after puberty. Signs of testicular torsion include intermittent pain, nausea, and vomiting. The exam reveals an enlarged, tender scrotum with scrotal edema (Oski & Johnson, 1997). Exam of the testes through Doppler ultrasound evidences blood flow to the testes and may aid in distinguishing torsion from other diagnoses.

315. **(D)** Recurrent abdominal pain (RAP) is a common entity that occurs in the school-age and adolescent population. It is characterized by vague, paroxysmal episodes of dull pain, located in the periumbilical or suprapubic regions. Autonomic symptoms may occur. It is defined by its chronic nature and is not associated with fatigue. Although it may interfere with normal activities, the pain should not awaken the child at night (Oberlander & Rappaport, 1993).

316. **(B)** Recurrent abdominal pain (RAP) occurs without a temporal association to meals, activity, or bowel habits. Although RAP can be associated with depression, psychologic factors have not been proven to be strongly associated with this entity (Oberlander & Rappaport, 1993). Obesity is not a risk factor to developing RAP, and heme-positive stools may be a sign of organic reasons for the pain and therefore should be investigated.

317. **(C)** In the absence of other positive findings, an appropriate evaluation of the child with chronic abdominal pain should include a CBC with differential, ESR, urinalysis, urine culture in females, and stool guaiac. Other diagnostics such as x-rays, throat cultures, liver function tests, and breath hydrogen tests should be reserved for children in whom history and physical exam reveal positive findings.

318. **(D)** The goal of treatment in RAP is to emphasize normality and encourage independence in dealing with the pain. The use of nonsteroidal antiinflammatory drugs (NSAIDs), as well as other medications, should be dis-

continued. Attempts should be made to lessen social attention and secondary gain that can be derived from the symptoms (Loening-Baucke, 1996).

319. **(C)** Left lower quadrant (LLQ) pain can be a manifestation of constipation, a common cause of persistent abdominal pain in children. Encopresis, the act of voluntary withholding of stool, can be associated with irritability, abdominal pain, distention, anorexia, and fecal soiling and requires a therapeutic regimen that involves disimpaction and behavioral regimens (Lewis & Ruldoph, 1997). Appendicitis typically causes right lower quadrant (RLQ) pain, cholethiasis causes right upper quadrant (RUQ) or periumbilical pain, and peptic ulcer disease causes epigastric discomfort.

320. **(A)** Hirschsprung's disease is a congenital abnormality that affects boys four times more often than girls and requires surgical intervention. In infants, the usual presentation of Hirschsprung's disease is constipation, an abdominal fecal mass, distention, vomiting, or diarrhea. The severity of symptoms is dependent on the degree of the abnormality. Severe cases can present in the newborn period as intestinal obstruction. Rectal prolapse, imperforate anus, and rectal bleeding are not frequently associated findings of Hirschsprung's disease (Milla, 1996).

321. **(C)** Encopresis is a more common condition than frequently recognized. Depending on the clinical study, the incidence is between 0.5 and 4% of the general population, occurring more frequently in boys than girls in a ratio approximating 4:1. While definitions vary from one researcher to another, consensus elements include an age > 4 years, duration of symptoms > 1 month, and soiling or involuntary defecation in inappropriate places (Howe & Walker, 1992).

322. **(A)** A careful and detailed history is the most important component in establishing the diagnosis of encopresis. A cursory history will often miss the abnormalities in bowel habits.

Parents and their children may be ashamed and fail to bring up the issue. In fact, parents are often unaware of the extent of the problem, especially with older children who are able to hide their symptoms (Schmitt, 1997). A physical exam is useful in ruling out medical conditions that may be differential diagnoses, including Hirschsprung's disease, hypothyroidism, and spinal defects. In the vast majority of cases the physical exam will be normal except for components relative to fecal retention. The inclusion of a rectal exam during the initial evaluation is a controversial issue, but is usually helpful in confirming the diagnosis. In children, in whom the rectal exam is perceived as overly intrusive, the exam can be deferred to follow-up visits or replaced by a flat plate of the abdomen to confirm the presence of excess stool. Additionally, an x-ray is often helpful in documenting progress in treatment. More intrusive diagnostic tests are rarely needed and should be reserved for refractory cases (Nolan & Oberklaid, 1993)

323. **(B)** The two common predisposing etiologies of encopresis include both behavioral and physiologic components (Schmitt, 1997). The behavioral component often includes oppositional behavior beginning during toddlerhood relating to toilet training and continuing into school age. Alternatively, attentional problems that lead the child to lose focus even on the daily routines of toileting are another common behavioral antecedent. The physiologic components have historically been thought to involve physiologic or nutritional constipation, but more recently have been recognized as inadequate rectal evacuation, abnormal anal tone, and rectal hyposensitivity (Nolan & Oberklaid, 1993). More significant structural abnormalities of the bowel have rarely, if ever, been associated with encopresis.

324. **(C)** The treatment of encopresis is best achieved through a combination of behavioral and medical management, including educating both the child and the parents about the physiologic components of the disease and the positive prognosis with appropriate therapy (Schmitt, 1997). Most children with encopresis have fecal backup requiring an adequate "cleaning out" before maintenance medication and behavioral approaches will be successful. Behavioral systems usually include a strategy for routine toilet time as well as a behavioral reward system. Though aversive behavior approaches have been attempted in the past, they have generally been found to be counterproductive and are rarely appropriate in current therapy.

325. **(D)** The prognosis in children with encopresis is generally quite positive with appropriate therapy. In fact, in excess of 60% have complete remission within 6 months and another 20–30% have much improvement. Approximately 10–20% tend to be more refractory and may need referral to specialty medical or psychological therapy (Nolan & Oberklaid, 1993). The prevalence of encopresis gradually decreases during the school-age years and is rarely reported in the adolescent child. Follow-up studies of children with a diagnosis of encopresis earlier in life do not seem to exhibit relapse beyond the age of puberty.

Genitourinary

CASES AND QUESTIONS

Questions 326–330

Four-year-old Britanny presents to your office today after her parent discovers an afternoon void to be grossly hematuric. Britanny has had no recent illness or rashes, although she did vomit once today after lunch. She, uncharacteristically, took an afternoon nap. There is no previous history of urinary tract infection. She is afebrile at this visit.

326. Your list of differential diagnoses for hematuria would include all of the following EXCEPT

   (A) Glomerulonephritis
   (B) Trauma
   (C) Benign recurrent hematuria
   (D) Inflammatory bowel disease

Britanny is alert and nontoxic appearing at this visit. Her physical examination is benign and there is no evidence of trauma. Blood pressure is 90/58. There is no gross edema.

327. Which of the following laboratory tests will help the PNP distinguish a lower urinary tract problem from an upper urinary tract problem?

   (A) + Leukocyte esterase on dipstick urine exam
   (B) Presence of urine casts
   (C) + RBCs and + protein
   (D) Presence of urine crystals

328. Which of following laboratory tests would be *most* helpful in helping to initially identify the cause of this 4-year-old's hematuria?

   (A) Clean-catch urine for microscopic examination
   (B) Renal ultrasound
   (C) Clean-catch urine for culture and sensitivities
   (D) VCUG

In reviewing Britanny's medical records, the PNP notes that she had a positive throat culture for group A beta-hemolytic streptococcus approximately 5 weeks ago, which was treated with penicillin VK for 10 days. Results of the macroscopic urinalysis today reveals 2+ blood, 2+ proteinuria, and + RBC casts.

329. The most likely cause of Britanny's hematuria is

   (A) Acute poststreptococcal glomerulonephritis
   (B) Hemolytic-uremic syndrome
   (C) Benign recurrent hematuria
   (D) Cystitis

330. A common physical finding in a child suspected to have acute poststreptococcal glomerulonephritis may include

   (A) Periorbital edema
   (B) Hypotension
   (C) Fever of 38.8°C (102°F) or greater
   (D) Hepatosplenomegaly

Questions 331–335

Jennifer is an 8-month-old female infant who presents to your clinic today with a 3-day history of mild upper respiratory infection. In addition, yesterday afternoon she developed a fever of 38.8°C (102°F) rectally, vomited once, and has been cranky since arising this morning. Appetite has been somewhat decreased today. She is alert and nontoxic appearing with no skin rashes and is well hydrated with a flat anterior fontanelle. There is no focus of infection on her physical examination except for clear nasal discharge. She attends day care twice a week, but the parents are unaware of any ill contacts at this time.

331. The primary presenting symptom of most infants and young children for urinary tract infections is

(A) Skin rash
(B) Fever
(C) Irritability
(D) Upper respiratory infection

In addition to obtaining a complete blood count with differential and blood culture for this infant with fever without source, the PNP will obtain a urine sample for culture and sensitivity.

332. The method of obtaining a urine culture in children has a major impact on the results. To avoid contamination of the urine, the sample should be obtained from this patient by which of the following methods?

(A) Clean-bag technique
(B) Clean-catch midstream specimen
(C) Urethral aspiration
(D) Bladder catheterization

The results of Jennifer's microscopic urinalysis are indicative of a urinary tract infection. She has a WBC count of 10,000. Urine and blood cultures are pending.

333. The most common causative organism for urinary tract infections in infants and children is

(A) Adenovirus
(B) *Shigella*
(C) *Escherichia coli*
(D) *Streptococcus pneumoniae*

Because Jennifer is nontoxic appearing and is able to tolerate oral fluids and medications at this time, she will be treated by the PNP with oral antibiotics on an outpatient basis pending urine and blood cultures.

334. Initial antibiotic therapy should be based on which of the following?

(A) Prior antibiotic history
(B) Severity of illness
(C) Child's age
(D) All of the above

335. In addition to at-home observation, fever control, and close telephone follow-up, management of this 8-month-old infant would include

1. Return for urine culture in 48 hours and again at end of 10-day course of oral antibiotics
2. No radiographic evaluation necessary because first urinary tract infection
3. Return for urine culture at end of 10-day course of oral antibiotics
4. Post-urinary tract infection radiographic evaluation following antibiotic treatment

(A) 3 and 4
(B) 2 and 3
(C) 1 and 2
(D) 1 and 4

Questions 336–338

Elizabeth is a 6-year-old female with acute onset dysuria. There has been no gross hematuria. She has been afebrile today, but her mother has noted increased frequency of urination and urgency over the past several days. There is no previous history of urinary tract infections and no recent illnesses over the past month. There has been no trauma, no abdominal pain, and no vomiting. PE findings are unremarkable and there is no CVA or abdominal tenderness.

336. Risk factors for urinary tract infections in children include all of the following EXCEPT

(A) Sexual abuse
(B) Poor perineal hygiene
(C) Circumcised penis
(D) Infrequent voiding

A clean-catch urine sample is obtained. Elizabeth's blood pressure is 88/60. Microscopic urinalysis is indicative of a urinary tract infection. Urine culture and sensitivity results are pending.

337. Optimal management of urinary tract infections in infants and children includes

   (A) Early diagnosis
   (B) Effective antibiotic treatment
   (C) Prevention of further infection
   (D) All of the above

338. Which of the following antibiotics is indicated in treating an uncomplicated urinary tract infection in an infant or child caused by a gram-negative bacteria such as *Escherichia coli?*

   (A) Amoxicillin
   (B) Trimethoprim-sulfamethoxazole
   (C) Nitrofurantoin
   (D) All of the above

Questions 339–340

Jody is an ill-appearing 17-year-old female who presents to your office today with complaints of dysuria, urinary frequency, and urgency. She has had these symptoms for 3 days and this afternoon after school developed a fever of 38.4°C (101.2°F) and abdominal pain at home. There has been no vomiting. There is no past or present history of sexual activity. On physical examination, there is diffuse abdominal tenderness over the suprapubic area and left-sided CVA tenderness.

339. Acute bacterial pyelonephritis

   (A) Almost never presents with frequency, urgency, and dysuria
   (B) Occurs only in sexually active adolescents
   (C) Follows the ascending route of urinary tract infections
   (D) Is characterized by urinary tract infection with fever over 37.7°C (100°F)

340. The most common causative organisms for urinary tract infections in adolescent girls include

   (A) *Pneumococcus, Escherichia coli, Enterococcus*
   (B) *Escherichia coli, Staphylococcus saprophyticus, Proteus mirabilis*
   (C) *Escherichia coli, Candida albicans, Shigella*
   (D) *Chlamydia trachomatis, Escherichia coli, Klebsiella*

Questions 341–343

Ben is a 12-year-old male who presents to your office today with sudden-onset scrotal swelling. He appears nontoxic; however, he is complaining of a significant amount of pain. He is afebrile with no history of recent illness and no history of scrotal trauma. He was last seen in your office 2 months ago for a pre-sports participation physical and received an MMR at that time.

341. Differential diagnosis for painful scrotal swelling would include all of the following EXCEPT

   (A) Testicular torsion
   (B) Epididymitis
   (C) Hydrocele
   (D) Hematocele secondary to trauma

Physical examination reveals a child with significant scrotal edema and unilateral tenderness. Pain does not disappear with elevation of the scrotum.

342. The most likely cause of this child's scrotal pain and edema is

   (A) Acute appendicitis
   (B) Mumps orchitis
   (C) Epididymitis
   (D) Torsion of the testis

343. The next step in management of this child with acute scrotal pain and edema should be

   (A) Rest, ice, and scrotal support
   (B) No intervention necessary at this time
   (C) Immediate surgical referral
   (D) 24-hour observation at home to observe change in scrotal size

Questions 344–346

Murray is a 14-year-old male who presents to your office today for a routine health assessment. A routine clean-catch urinalysis is obtained during this visit. The laboratory report reveals 2+ proteinuria with no hematuria. Physical examination findings were entirely unremarkable and there is no evidence of edema. There have been no recent illnesses or medication use and he is afebrile with BP 100/70.

344. The most likely cause of this 14-year-old's proteinuria is

(A) Acute nephritic syndrome
(B) Orthostatic proteinuria
(C) Exercise-induced proteinuria
(D) Fever-induced proteinuria

345. The next most likely step in management of this 14-year-old's proteinuria would be

(A) Immediate hospitalization and evaluation
(B) 24-hour urine collection for protein
(C) No evaluation necessary at this time as child is asymptomatic
(D) Obtaining two timed urine samples for urinalysis

346. Which of the following statements regarding orthostatic proteinuria is *true?*

(A) Studies have shown a significant increase in the incidence of renal disease.
(B) It is associated with an increased risk of hypertension in adulthood.
(C) Studies have shown no increase in the incidence of renal disease.
(D) It is an uncommon finding in children and adolescents.

Questions 347–349

Luis is a 2-week-old male who reports for a well-child examination. He is a breast-fed infant with excellent health and weight gain. He was a full-term infant of a para 3, gravida 3 mother. To date, he has received one HBV vaccine. During today's physical examination the PNP notes an undescended right testicle. The left testicle is fully palpable. He is uncircumcised, with normal uretheral opening and urine stream.

347. All the following statements regarding cryptorchidism are true EXCEPT

(A) It is thought to occur secondary to decreased testosterone levels
(B) 80% will spontaneously descend into the scrotum by age 1 year
(C) Surgical orchidopexy remains the standard treatment
(D) It only occurs unilaterally

348. The most appropriate management of this infant's cryptorchidism is

(A) Explanation and reassurance to parents with follow-up at next scheduled well-child examination at age 2 months
(B) Referral to urologist
(C) Refer for possible treatment with human chorionic gonadotropin (hCG)
(D) None of the above

349. Luis's parents have questions regarding care of his uncircumcised penis. The most appropriate advice is

(A) No forcible retraction of the foreskin
(B) Forcibly retract the foreskin qd
(C) Gentle retraction of the foreskin with each diaper change to loosen adhesions
(D) None of the above

ANSWERS AND RATIONALES

326. **(D)** The list of differential diagnosis of hematuria is extensive. The most common causes seen in clinical practice include urinary tract infection (bacterial and viral), trauma (kidney, bladder, external), benign recurrent hematuria, and glomerulonephritis (Norman, 1997).

327. **(B)** When evaluating a child for hematuria, it should be determined whether the bleeding is originating in the upper or the lower urinary tract. Upper urinary tract bleeding would most likely present with the following: no clots, RBC casts, brown or cola-color urine, > 2+ proteinuria. Lower urinary tract bleeding would most likely present with the following: clots, bright red urine, < 2+ proteinuria, no RBC casts.

328. **(A)** Clean-catch urine for microscopic examination would be most helpful in initially identifying the cause of this 4-year-old child's hematuria. Examination of urine sediment is the key in initiating a workup for hematuria. Pyuria suggests a bacterial infection and a urine culture should be obtained. Glomerular hematuria is manifested by the presence of RBC casts or > 2+ proteinuria, or both.

329. **(A)** A typical presentation of poststreptococcal glomerulonephritis is a child who has sudden onset of brown or grossly bloody urine 1–3 weeks following a sore throat. Benign recurrent hematuria is an idiopathic disorder typically occurring in an asymptomatic child. The hematuria is usually microscopic and subsides over time. There may be a positive family history of similar symptoms. Cystitis usually presents with symptoms of dysuria, urgency, and frequency, usually without fever. Hemolytic-uremic syndrome (HUS) is one of the most common causes of acute renal failure in children under 2 years of age. It is a multisystem disorder due to infection with *E. coli* 157:07. Gross hematuria is an uncommon finding in HUS (Cronan & Norman, 1995).

330. **(A)** Clinically, with acute post-streptococcal glomerulonephritis, a child can have smokey, red, or tea-colored urine 1–3 weeks following a sore throat. Urine output may be decreased and edema, most commonly periorbital, may be present. The child may be entirely asymptomatic or very ill depending on the amount of renal involvement at the time of examination.

331. **(B)** Fever is the most common symptom in infants less than 1 year of age. Symptoms of urinary tract infections in young infants are usually nonspecific and may include vomiting, poor feeding, or irritability. Other less common findings in young infants may include jaundice, abdominal pain, and sepsis. It is important to examine an infant's growth curve because children with frequent urinary tract infections or renal problems may have a decreased growth rate. Failure to thrive is not uncommon among infants with urinary tract infections.

332. **(D)** Bladder catherization would be the preferred method for obtaining a urine culture in this 8-month-old infant. Urine specimens obtained using clean-bag technique should not be sent for urine culture because of their high rate for contamination. A clean-catch midstream specimen, a specimen obtained by bladder catheterization, or one obtained by suprapubic aspiration are the preferred methods of obtaining a urine sample for culture.

333. **(C)** Urinary tract infections are usually caused by bacteria that ascend up the urethra into the bladder. *Escherichia coli* is the most common organism associated with urinary tract infections. Other common pathogens include *Enterobacter, Klebsiella, Proteus* species, and enterococci. Cystitis may also be caused by adenovirus.

334. **(D)** Initial antimicrobial treatment should be based on prior antibiotic history, severity of symptoms, child's age, and response to initial antibiotic therapy (Leonard & Shaw, 1997; Todd, 1995).

335. **(D)** A repeat urine culture should be obtained after 48 hours of treatment to ensure that the urine is sterile and then repeated after a 10-day course of oral antibiotics. The goal of renal imaging is to evaluate the entire urinary tract. The first urinary tract infections in all boys and in girls less than 3 years of age should be radiographically evaluated with a voiding cystourethrogram, renal ultrasound, and renal cortical scan (DMSA) (Heldrich, 1995).

336. **(C)** In infancy, prevalence of urinary tract infections in both females and males (usually uncircumcised) is fairly equal. Beginning in late infancy and childhood, UTI is more common in females than males. Risk factors for urinary tract infections in females include infrequent voiding, constipation, frequent use of bubble bath, sexual abuse, pinworms, and poor perineal hygiene. Urologic abnormalities, indwelling uretheral catheterization, and neurogenic bladder are risk factors for both males and females.

337. **(D)** Early identification, treatment, prevention, and radiographic evaluation of urinary tract infections in young children is essential to prevent pyelonephritis and/or chronic renal infections, which may eventually lead to renal damage or renal scarring.

338. **(D)** The choice of antibiotic for treatment of urinary tract infection should first be verified by urine culture and sensitivity. For uncomplicated cases of urinary tract infection caused by a single gram-negative such as *E. coli*, a single oral antibiotic such as amoxicillin, trimethoprim-sulfamethoxazole, or nitrofurantoin can be initiated for a 10-day course (Leonard & Shaw, 1997; Todd, 1995).

339. **(C)** Acute bacterial pyelonephritis is an inflammation of the kidneys and ureters. It is most commonly caused by bacteria that have ascended from the bladder after entering through the urethra. It is characterized by a sudden-onset fever and chills with dull pain in the flank over one or both kidneys. Usually there are associated signs of cystitis including urinary frequency, urgency with burning, and pyuria.

340. **(B)** Common pathogens in community-acquired urinary tract infections in adolescents include *E. coli* and *P. mirabilis.* In addition, adolescent girls may have symptoms of cystitis from low colony counts of *S. saprophyticus* (Leonard & Shaw, 1997).

341. **(C)** Testicular torsion is a twisting of the spermatic cord resulting in sudden, unilateral testicular pain with swelling and tenderness. Gentle lifting of the testes does not relieve pain. The child may have fever and vomiting and there are no associated urinary tract symptoms. Epididymitis is an inflammation of the epididymis resulting in sudden, unilateral testicular pain with erythema, swelling, and tenderness. Unlike the case of testicular torsion, gentle lifting of the scrotum decreases testicular pain. Associated symptoms include dysuria, fever, chills, and urinary frequency. Testicular trauma usually results from direct trauma to the scrotum, which appears tender, swollen, and bruised. Hydrocele is a nontender swelling of the scrotum due to collection of peritoneal fluid. Scrotal skin is normal and the hydrocele is occasionally associated with an accompanying hernia.

342. **(D)** Based on this child's health history and physical examination, the most likely cause of his unilateral scrotal pain is testicular torsion. Orchitis, or inflammation of the testis, presents with swelling, tenderness, and pain of the scrotum accompanied by fever, chills, and urinary symptoms. Elevating the scrotum decreases the pain. The most common cause of orchitis in prepubertal males is mumps.

343. **(C)** Testicular torsion is a surgical emergency and should be immediately referred for surgical evaluation. Continued torsion of the testis may result in gangrene and/or loss of the testis.

344. **(B)** Proteinuria is a common finding in children. It is often discovered on a routine urinalysis and is thought to be the cause of up to 30% of proteinurias on random routine urinalysis. The child excretes abnormal amounts of urinary protein when in the upright position, but excretes normal amounts of urinary protein when lying flat. Exercise-induced and fever-induced proteinuria are also benign, though less common, causes of proteinuria on random routine urinalysis. Acute nephritic syndrome is associated with hematuria, red blood cell casts, systemic hypertension, and edema.

345. **(D)** Orthostatic proteinuria can be diagnosed by obtaining two timed urine collections, one from the recumbent position and then one from a standing position.

346. **(C)** Studies that have followed children and adolescents with orthostatic proteinuria have documented normal renal function in all patients in whom renal function was normal at the outset of the initial finding of proteinuria (Langman, 1993).

347. **(D)** Cryptorchidism, or undescended testis, may be unilateral (most common) or bilateral. It is thought to occur secondary to decreased testosterone levels. Eighty percent of cases of cryptorchidism will spontaneously descend into the scrotum by age 1 year. Administration of human chorionic gonadotropin (hCG) has been used with some success in Europe as an alternative to surgery. However, in the United States, surgical orchidopexy remains the standard treatment in cases where the testis does not spontaneously descend by age 1–2 years (Tarry, 1997).

348. **(A)** It is thought that 80% of all cases of undescended testis will spontaneously descend in the first year of life. Therefore, appropriate management for this child would be explanation and reassurance to parents with follow-up at next scheduled well-child examination at age 2 months.

349. **(A)** As the normal foreskin is adherent to the glans during the first year of life, no special care is required for the male infant with an uncircumcised penis. The foreskin is nonretractable in 80% of male infants at age 6 months and 10% at age 3 years. Forceable retraction of the foreskin is painful and may lead to rupture of the glans-foreskin adhesions, causing a phimosis (Tarry, 1997).

Gynecologic

CASES AND QUESTIONS

CASES AND QUESTIONS

Questions 350–354

Carol is a 17-year-old honors student at the local high school. She is accompanied on this visit by her mother, who is worried because her daughter has been complaining about back pain that kept her up all night. Carol states the pain began yesterday and now feels worse. She states she didn't hurt herself or "anything" like that. She states she otherwise feels fine. She appears quiet and withdrawn and will not make eye contact. She has no drug allergies and has otherwise been a healthy young woman with no major illnesses. She has not tried any OTC medication and is on no other medication at this time. Her mother decides to wait in the waiting room.

350. "Teen dating violence" describes a relationship in which one partner exerts power and control over another through physical violence, emotional abuse, economic control, and/or sexual abuse. A pattern of coercion often keeps the participants in this situation. Many teens mistake jealousy and control for love. The underlying reason for violence includes

  (A) Child abuse
  (B) Depression
  (C) Drug and alcohol abuse
  (D) All of the above

351. Carol is quiet but will answer some questions. She is guarded when you try to evaluate her back. Examination of the middle and lower back reveals several ecchymotic areas with some swelling. What would be your best response?

  (A) "Oh my. You must have fallen on something. Don't you remember?"
  (B) "You said you didn't hurt yourself, but how did you get these bruises?"
  (C) "You know, Carol, when I've seen bruises like this before, it's because someone was being hurt by someone else. Did somebody hit you or hurt you?"
  (D) "I have to report this because I'm a mandated reporter."

352. Carol now tells you that her boyfriend did this to her and it was her fault because she was late picking him up from work. Which of the following responses would *not* be appropriate?

  (A) "Why were you so late?"
  (B) "There is nothing you could have done to warrant being hurt like this."
  (C) "I'm concerned for your safety."
  (D) "Have incidents like this happened before?"

353. Carol tells you that her boyfriend is always hitting her, calling her names, and putting her down. She states she had tried to break up with him but he won't let her. Additional information that is important to ask includes

  (A) "Does he use drugs or alcohol?"
  (B) "Has he ever been in trouble with the police?"
  (C) "Do you think he is capable of carrying out his threats?"
  (D) All of the above

354. Carol tells you she doesn't know what to do and that she hasn't told her parents because she doesn't want them to be disappointed in her. She states she has a "great" relationship with her parents and has always been able to talk to her mom—but she just wanted to take care of this on her own. Your best advice now would be

    (A) "You need to tell your mother and if you don't, I'm going to have to."

    (B) "Have you thought about doing some counseling with your boyfriend?"

    (C) "I understand what you are saying and I'm worried about your safety. I bet your mom would want to know and could help you figure out what was the safest thing to do."

    (D) None of the above

Questions 355–359

Heather is a 19-year-old gravida 1, para 1 who presents to the clinic today with nausea, stomach discomfort, and great fatigue. She states these symptoms began 3–4 days ago and she is not feeling any better. She denies fever, diarrhea, and dysuria and states that no one else at home is ill. She has vomited three times over the past 4 days, always in the morning. She states she has no appetite. She last received Depo-Provera 18 weeks ago and is not on any other medication.

355. Based on the information given in the history, which of the following diagnoses is most likely?

    (A) Gastroenteritis

    (B) Adverse reaction to Depo-Provera

    (C) Early pregnancy

    (D) Viral syndrome

356. Heather is afebrile. Her HEENT exam is within normal limits. You continue to assess her by asking questions related to her reproductive health. Which of the following questions would you ask *first*?

    (A) When was your last Pap smear?

    (B) Have you ever had a sexually transmitted disease?

    (C) Do you think you are pregnant?

    (D) When was your last menstrual period?

357. Heather provides you with more history. She states that while she was on Depo for the past year, her periods were very irregular and thus she decided to stop. She received her last dose 18 weeks ago and was waiting for a period so she could start the pill. Her last menstrual period was 3 months ago and it was not "normal." She is sexually active with the father of her child, is monogamous, and believes he is also. They use condoms every time, except maybe once. Your best response to her is

    (A) "Do you feel like you are pregnant?"

    (B) "Well, it sounds to me like you are pregnant. What do you plan to do?"

    (C) "I'm not sure what is causing you to feel this way, so I'll run a few tests."

    (D) "Since condoms aren't as effective as Depo, you probably should have stayed on it."

358. You want to rule out that Heather is pregnant. Which of the following is a *true* statement?

    (A) Only the tests that identify the beta subunit are specific for human chorionic gonadotropin (hCG) hormone.

    (B) hCG levels in normal pregnancy rise predictably, doubling approximately every 1–2 days during the first 30 days of gestation.

    (C) False-positive tests result from cross-reactions with luteinizing hormone (LH).

    (D) All of the above.

359. The positive signs of pregnancy include

    (A) Palpation of fetal parts

    (B) Changes in uterine size, shape, and consistency

    (C) Positive fetal heart rate

    (D) Abdominal enlargement

Questions 360–363

Carrie is a 15-year-old Caucasian female who is concerned about cramping during her menses. Carrie states she has never engaged in sexual intercourse, adding, "I'm not ready for that yet." She has never had a pelvic exam. She states that she has no abnormal discharge or odor and that her periods have been regular every month for the past 2 years. Menarche occurred at age 13. Carrie states that the last two cycles have caused her to miss work and school. She also reports that her cramps began 1 year after the onset of her menses. During the last two cycles, the cramps began a few hours before flow and lasted 2–3 days once flow began. She has used over-the-counter (OTC) medication with little relief.

360. The most likely diagnosis for Carrie would be

(A) Secondary dysmenorrhea
(B) Endometriosis
(C) Primary dysmenorrhea
(D) Pelvic inflammatory disease

361. An etiology for Carrie's symptoms includes

(A) Subserosal myomata
(B) Ovarian cyst
(C) Cervical stenosis
(D) Spasms

362. There are many other symptoms associated with dysmenorrhea. All the following are correct EXCEPT

(A) Hematuria
(B) Severe headaches
(C) Backache
(D) Diarrhea or constipation

363. Which of the following are treatments for dysmenorrhea?

(A) Ibuprofen (Motrin) 400 mg, 1 qid with a loading dose of 800–1200 mg
(B) Mefenamic acid (Ponstel) 550 mg, 2 stat then 1 q6h
(C) Anaprox 250 mg q8h
(D) All of the above

Questions 364–367

Mrs. Jones' 5-year-old daughter Claire complains of vaginal discharge, pain on urination, redness, and pruritus. Mrs. Jones reports that Claire needs to change her underwear 3–4 times per day and that this has been going on for the past 3 weeks. She describes a thick, white, sometimes yellowish discharge. Mrs. Jones states that she does not observe Claire washing or using the bathroom. She further states that Claire prefers to take a bath with bubble bath. Claire also is very active with dancing and gymnastics. She has not been on antibiotics lately and her 3-year-old brother has been ill with "a respiratory infection." Claire has no known drug allergies and takes a multivitamin (Flintstones) every day.

364. Causes of vulvovaginitis in a prepubescent child include all the following EXCEPT

(A) Anatomic abnormality
(B) Tight fitting clothes
(C) Bubble baths and harsh soaps
(D) Respiratory, enteric, or sexually transmitted pathogens

365. The history should include

(A) Information about a recent upper respiratory infection in the patient or a family member
(B) Hygiene habits
(C) Questions that may elicit a history of sexual abuse
(D) All of the above

366. The differential diagnosis for prepubescent vulvovaginitis includes all the following EXCEPT

(A) Foreign body
(B) Leukorrhea
(C) Sexual abuse
(D) Pinworms

367. The physical exam reveals a scanty mucoid discharge and an erythematous introitus. The hymen is redundant and symmetrical. The rectal exam is normal as well. The initial treatment for Claire would include

(A) Scheduling Claire for a gynecologic exam under anesthesia
(B) The use of white cotton underwear front-to-back wiping, loose fitting clothes, and nylon tights
(C) No bubble baths, switching to soaps like Basis, Dove, or Neutrogena, with no soap to the vulva
(D) Amoxicillin 250 mg tid for 10 days

Questions 368–373

Julia is an 18-year-old senior in high school who plans to attend college next year. She states she has had a vaginal discharge on and off since her menses ended 1 week ago. Her menses came on time and lasted 4 days. She states the discharge is white and thick and that every time she wipes, there are copious amounts. Julia is sexually active with a 20-year-old boyfriend. This is her only lifetime partner and she reports that he has had at least two other partners. She is on oral contraception and uses condoms every time. She has not missed any pills. Julia states that the last time she had intercourse (2 weeks ago), she bled after. Her gynecologic exam 3 months ago revealed a normal Pap smear with negative cervical cultures for chlamydia and gonorrhea.

368. In obtaining a history from Julia, which of the following questions about her symptoms are important?

(A) The presence of erythema
(B) The color, onset, odor, and consistency of the discharge
(C) Recent treatment with antibiotics
(D) All of the above

369. On physical exam you inspect the external genitalia for

(A) Friability
(B) Lesions, erythema, edema, and excoriations
(C) Ectropion
(D) All of the above

370. The differential diagnosis includes all of the following EXCEPT

(A) Normal physiologic discharge
(B) Herpes simplex
(C) Molluscum contagiosum
(D) Condylomata

371. Which is the most common organism found in normal vaginal flora?

(A) Lactobacillus
(B) Streptococci

(C) Mycoplasma
(D) *Gardnerella vaginalis*

372. Having examined Julia, you find that her wet mount is normal. You have obtained cultures to rule out a sexually transmitted disease (STD) as well as a vaginal culture. Her vaginal pH is 3.8. There are no lesions present and her bimanual exam was within normal limits. Your recommendations for Julia include all of the following EXCEPT

(A) Education about personal hygiene
(B) Aci-jel cream qhs for 1 week
(C) Antibiotics for 7 days
(D) Return to the clinic in 2 weeks if no improvement

373. Predisposing factors that may cause vaginitis include which of the following?

(A) Pregnancy
(B) Diabetes mellitus
(C) Immunosuppression
(D) All of the above

Questions 374–379

Mrs. Harris brings her 15-year-old daughter Kelly to the clinic today. Kelly started her menses at age 12 years, but it stopped 7 months ago. She's worried because Kelly keeps a busy schedule, doesn't always eat well, and only gets 6–7 hours of sleep each night. Mrs. Harris further states that she is concerned as her 28-year-old sister died of ovarian cancer. When you meet with Kelly, she tells you that she is a gymnast and runs 3–4 miles per day, 5 days out of the week. She states she has never had intercourse and uses no drugs.

374. This type of amenorrhea is most likely

(A) Primary amenorrhea
(B) Normal
(C) Secondary amenorrhea
(D) Turner's syndrome

375. Primary amenorrhea is associated with which of the following syndromes?

    (A) Kallmann's syndrome, Rokitansky-Küster-Hauser syndrome, Turner's syndrome
    (B) Horner's syndrome, Cushing's syndrome, Stein-Leventhal syndrome
    (C) Turner's syndrome, Prader-Willi syndrome, Klinefelter's syndrome
    (D) Adrenocortical hyperplasia syndrome, Down syndrome, Gardner's syndrome

376. The etiology for secondary amenorrhea includes which of the following?

    (A) Pregnancy, pituitary tumor, rapid weight gain
    (B) Rapid weight loss, excessive exercise, thyroid disease
    (C) Anorexia, Asherman's syndrome, too little body fat
    (D) All of the above

377. Physical exam should include which of the following?

    (A) Patient's weight, exam of the thyroid, breast exam, vaginal exam
    (B) HEENT, breasts, vaginal exam
    (C) Abdominal exam, breast exam, rectovaginal exam
    (D) Complete head-to-toe examination

378. Laboratory evaluation should include which of the following?

    (A) Prolactin level
    (B) TSH, FSH, LH
    (C) Dehydroepiandrosterone sulfate (DHAS)
    (D) All of the above

379. If test results are all within normal limits, your treatment should be

    (A) Medroxyprogesterone acetate (Provera) 35 mg for 7 days
    (B) Start oral contraceptives
    (C) Give a shot of Depo-Provera 150 mg IM
    (D) Provera 10 mg for 5 days

Questions 380–383

Janeen is a 23-year-old single, working female who presents to the clinic today complaining of a "bump" on the outside of her vagina and feeling fatigued. She complains of dyspareunia and states that the fatigue has been ongoing for the past 3–4 days. She reports urinary frequency with pain, and feels the urge to void even after voiding. Over the last few days, she reports feeling feverish, although she has not taken her temperature. Janeen is on Ortho-Novum 1/35 and has not missed any pills. She reports no drug allergies. Her LMP was 2 weeks ago. She has had a new partner for the past 3 months and is not using condoms. She has a history of abnormal Pap smears, and had colposcopy and biopsies 3 months ago that were consistent with human papilloma virus, although she states she has never seen an external lesion. She denies any other sexually transmitted diseases (STDs). She has not asked her partner if he has any symptoms. Janeen always keeps her appointments and follows her treatment plans.

380. As you hear this history, you consider which of the following as the possible diagnosis?

    (A) Urinary tract infection
    (B) Urinary tract infection and chlamydia
    (C) Herpes
    (D) All of the above

381. On physical examination, you note the following: three vesicular lesions containing cloudy liquid, surrounded by an erythematous base on the left labia majora, and two small ulcerative lesions with irregular borders aligned on the right labia majora. The patient also has mild bilateral inguinal adenopathy. The patient states that the pain is severe when examined. Based on these findings your differential diagnosis is

    (A) Herpes simplex virus (HSV), syphilis, chancroid, granuloma inguinale
    (B) HSV, UTI, syphilis, gonorrhea (Gc)
    (C) UTI, chancroid, HSV, *Chlamydia trachomatis*
    (D) Syphilis, HSV, HPV (human papilloma virus)

382. Janeen is very uncomfortable with the external exam and states she doesn't wish to have a speculum exam. Your next course of action would be

(A) Tell her that she needs to have the speculum exam and that you know she is uncomfortable, but you will be gentle and it won't take long.

(B) Apply xylocaine gel to the external genitalia, then conduct the speculum exam obtaining cultures for HSV, Gc, chlamydia.

(C) Scrape the lesions for virology cultures, defer the speculum exam, and treat the patient for Gc, chlamydia, and HSV.

(D) Scrape the lesions for virology cultures, begin to treat with acyclovir, and have the patient return in 3–4 days for a speculum exam. Obtain a urine culture and rapid plasma reagent (RPR) and stress to the patient the importance of returning for continuing evaluation and treatment.

383. Three days later the viral culture returns positive for HSV type II. The urine culture grows out greater than 100,000 of *E. coli.* Your next course of action is

(A) Continue on acyclovir 500 mg bid, po for 2 weeks

(B) Continue on acyclovir 200 mg po 5 times/day for another 1–2 weeks, or until clinical resolution is attained

(C) Bactrim double strength, one tab po bid for 7 days while continuing on acyclovir 200 mg po 5 times/day for 4–7 days more, or until clinical resolution is attained

(D) Have the patient continue on acyclovir 500 mg po for 2 weeks, as that will also cover the UTI

ANSWERS AND RATIONALES

350. **(D)** Many women who present with depression are in fact living in a violent home. If the patient is not routinely screened for partner violence, a victim may not disclose. Many victims of domestic abuse start using drugs and alcohol as a means of self-medicating. Teens who present with injuries may be subjected to abuse by a parent, caretaker, boyfriend, or girlfriend. Often, when a victim is attacked, the perpetrator makes threats to assure that the victim will keep the secret (Lewis-O'Connor, 1997; Kerouac et al., 1986).

351. **(C)** It is important not to sound accusatory and to try to ask open-ended questions while projecting sincerity and concern. Threatening to report will generally result in the patient's withdrawing from the interview and making no further disclosure. The goal is to help the patient disclose, making her feel safe with the examiner (Lewis-O'Connor, 1997).

352. **(A)** Avoid victim-blaming statements. Asking the patient why she was so late implies that she deserved the beating. Informing her that violence is not acceptable, and is in fact criminal, and that nothing she did warrants physical violence, puts the responsibility on the perpetrator. Letting her know you're concerned for her safety helps her to see that she is in danger. Asking open-ended questions about other incidents helps you and the patient assess how lethal the situation is (Lewis-O'Connor, 1997; Campbell & Humphreys, 1993).

353. **(D)** Stating that it is not her fault puts the blame where it belongs: on the perpetrator. Asking about drugs and alcohol and involvement with the police begins to assess how volatile and dangerous her situation is. Asking such questions assesses her risk. Once this information is available, start to develop a safety plan with the patient (Lewis-O'Connor, 1997).

354. **(C)** Start to to empower the client by helping her problem-solve and identify resources that may assist her in making decisions. Couples counseling is contraindicated when there is violence in a relationship; in fact, it may put a woman in further harm's way. Threatening to tell her mother will only isolate the patient from you (Lewis-O'Connor, 1997).

355. **(C)** The likelihood of gastroenteritis is low with no diarrhea and no complaint of abdominal cramping. Since the last shot of Depo-Provera was 18 months ago, it is unlikely that the contraceptive is causing her current problems. This leaves a 19-year-old woman who has not had a Depo injection within the last 18 weeks, who has nausea and vomiting in the morning. The symptoms described in the history lead you to suspect an early pregnancy (Neimstein, 1984; Starr et al., 1995).

356. **(D)** While it is important to assess for abnormal Pap smears and sexually transmitted diseases in a postpubescent female, you must always ask the date of her last menstrual period (LMP). A pregnancy test in situations like this is a must. Questions relating to LMP and the possibility of pregnancy provide the clinician with the opportunity to discuss this important topic with young women (Beck, 1993).

357. **(A)** Answer B is presumptive and not very helpful at this point. Responding with D implies that the patient made a bad choice, which is not true. And while C is a good choice, A begins to assess the patient's thinking and provides information about her readiness to accept pregnancy.

358. **(D)** Modern tests are based on the detection of human chorionic gonadotropin (hCG) in a woman's blood or urine. In a normal pregnancy, hCG rises predictably, doubling approximately every 1–2 days during the first 30 days of gestation. hCG contains a beta subunit. These beta subunits are almost identical to LH, FSH, and TSH. Thus, pregnancy tests that detect the beta subunit can produce false-positive tests (Lichtman & Papera, 1990).

359. **(C)** The *positive* signs of pregnancy include: fetal heart rate, perception of fetal movement by a person other than the patient, or sonographic evidence of a fetus. The *probable* signs of pregnancy include: abdominal enlargement, changes in uterine size, shape, consistency, Braxton Hicks contractions, and palpation of fetal parts (Frederickson & Wilkins-Haug, 1991).

360. **(C)** Secondary dysmenorrhea is painful menstruation due to an identifiable pathologic or iatrogenic condition, readily identifiable on the basis of the history and the findings in a physical exam. Patients with endometriosis report cyclic and acyclic pelvic pain, with some experiencing an increase in symptoms midcycle. The pain may increase in severity over time and may be present throughout the month. Other symptoms associated with endometriosis include dysmenorrhea, painful defecation, dyspareunia, irregular bleeding, and spotting. Pelvic inflammatory disease (PID) is a chronic or acute infectious process within the pelvic cavity that may or may not be associated with menses. Patients often complain of fever, chills, increase in vaginal discharge, and heavier than usual menses. Primary dysmenorrhea is the occurrence of painful menses beginning within several years of menarche and in the absence of any pelvic pathology. Primary dysmenorrhea is classified as congestive or spasmodic according to symptoms, cause, and treatment (Hawkins et a1., 1993; Emans & Goldstein, 1990).

361. **(D)** Subserosal myomatas, ovarian cysts, and cervical stenosis are extrauterine causes associated with secondary dysmenorrhea. Spasmodic dysmenorrhea is often the most debilitating of menstrual discomforts. It occurs as the result of ovulation and the production of prostaglandins. These cause an increase in myometrial contractions and constriction of small endometrial blood vessels, with subsequent tissue ischemia, endometrial disintegration, bleeding, and pain (Hawkins et al., 1993).

362. **(A)** Hematuria is not a symptom associated with dysmenorrhea (Hawkins et al., 1993). Should a patient present with dysmenorrhea, and incidentally have hematuria, the patient should also have a workup for hematuria.

363. **(A)** The most common approach to the treatment of dysmenorrhea is to prescribe a nonsteroidal antiinflammatory (NSAID) compound. Common medications for the treatment of dysmenorrhea are ibuprofen, 400 mg every 4–6 hours to 800 mg 3 times a day, with a loading dose of 800–1200 mg; mefenamic acid (Ponstel) 250 mg, with a 500-mg loading dose, and 250 mg every 6 hours; or Anaprox 550 mg twice a day, or a 500-mg loading dose, and 275 mg every 6 hours (Emans & Goldstein, 1990; Hawkins et al., 1993).

364. **(A)** Because of poor hygiene, the location of the vagina and anus, the lack of protective hairs, labial fat pads, and the lack of estrogenization, the vulvar skin is susceptible to irritation and is easily affected by medication, clothing, and pathogens. Vaginal cultures frequently grow lactobacilli, diphtheroids, *Staphylococcus epidermidis*, or streptococci. Also seen are gram-negative enteric pathogens, such as *Escherichia coli*, *Shigella*, and *Yersinia*. Either a hymenal opening that does not allow normal vaginal drainage or a gaping hymenal ring that allows easy contamination of the vagina can predispose a child to a nonspecific vaginitis. The presence of a sexually transmitted disease strongly suggests sexual abuse. Restrictive clothes and the use of soaps may serve as an irritant causing vaginitis (Emans & Goldstein, 1990).

365.   **(D)** A history of recent infection in the patient or in a family member is important, as a streptococcal respiratory infection may lead to a vaginitis. Overvigorous cleansing of the vulva and poor habits related to wiping and the wearing of tight-fitting clothes also can lead to vaginitis (Emans & Goldstein, 1990). Eliciting a history of abuse can be difficult but not impossible and is critical so that an abused child does not go undetected (Lewis-O'Connor et al., 1995).

366.   **(B)** A foul-smelling discharge often is a sign of a foreign body in the vagina, such as toilet paper (Emans & Goldstein, 1990) or small objects such as toys. Leukorrhea is physiologic and should not be confused with vulvovaginitis. Newborns and pubescent girls often have copious secretions secondary to the effect of estrogen on the vaginal mucosa. In newborns, this disappears 2–3 weeks after birth. Pinworms are responsible for vulvar and rectal pruritis (Emans & Goldstein, 1990). Children with vulvovaginitis may have been sexually abused. Pathogens consistent with a sexually transmitted disease may be detected as well as a history of fondling, digital penetration, or intercourse (Lewis-O'Connor et al., 1995).

367.   **(C)** Scheduling Claire for an exam under general anesthesia at this point is not necessary. Should Claire show persistent, purulent, or recurrent vaginal discharge with no response to treatment, and if the clinician is unable to visualize the cervix or vagina, a more thorough evaluation would be warranted. Nylon tights should be avoided and antibiotic therapy should only be prescribed when an organism has been detected (Emans & Goldstein, 1990).

368.   **(B)** A description of the discharge should include color, onset, odor, consistency, constant versus intermittent, and color of discharge on underwear (Hawkins et al., 1993). Erythema is not a term used to describe discharge.

369.   **(B)** When inspecting the external genitalia you should be looking for erythema, excoriations, lesions, and edema. The vaginal/speculum exam includes observation of a foreign body (ie, tampon), erythema and edema of the vagina as well as inspection of the cervix for erythema, erosion, ectropion, friability, serous sanguineous discharge, or lesions (Hawkins et al., 1993).

370.   **(C)** Molluscum contagiosum is an infectious disease of the skin caused by a member of the poxvirus group. Lesions affect the face, arms, genitals, abdomen, and thighs. The patient usually presents with a complaint of painless "bumps," which are fleshy growths (Hawkins et al., 1993). Patients are usually asymptomatic (Neimstein, 1984).

371.   **(A)** Lactobacillus, an aerobic gram-positive rod, is the most common bacteria found in the vagina of both symptomatic and asymptomatic females. Other bacterial flora include streptococci, staphylococci, diphtheroids, *Gardnerella vaginalis, E. coli,* and several anaerobic organisms. *Candida* and *Mycoplasma* species are also commonly found (Frederickson & Wilkins-Haug, 1991).

372.   **(C)** There is no need to treat with an antibiotic unless a pathogen has been identified or unless the physical exam reveals clinical data that supports treatment (Hawkins et al., 1993).

373.   **(D)** Strong evidence exists that vaginal infections are a result of certain predisposing factors that include diabetes mellitus, pregnancy, oral contraceptive use, steroids, antibiotic therapy (Neimstein, 1984) as well as menstruation and immunosuppression.

374.   **(C)** Secondary amenorrhea is the cessation of menses after it has been established at puberty, while primary amenorrhea is the failure of menses to occur at puberty (Hawkins et al., 1993). The incidence of primary amenorrhea is less than 0.1%, and 0.7% for secondary amenorrhea (Frederickson & Wilkins-Haug, 1991).

375. **(A)** Turner's syndrome, or gonadal failure, accounts for one-third of all patients with primary amenorrhea (Frederickson & Wilkins-Haug, 1991). Those with Turner's are of short stature with widely spaced nipples, webbed neck, low hairline, short fourth or fifth metacarpals, cubitus valgus, ptosis, low-set ears, narrow, high arched palates, lymphedema, and multiple pigmented nevi (Emans & Goldstein, 1990). Kallmann's syndrome causes primary amenorrhea that results from inadequate levels of GnRH and anosmia. These patients have infantile sexual development (Frederickson & Wilkins-Haug, 1991). Rokitansky-Küster-Hauser syndrome is a mullerian anomaly that results in uterovaginal agenesis, which accounts for 20% of primary amenorrhea cases. Congenital adrenocortical hyperplasia is a condition most commonly seen in female newborns. The condition varies from labial fusion with or without clitoromegaly to a "male phallus" with labial fusion and rugae on the labioscrotal folds (Emans & Goldstein, 1990). These cases are usually diagnosed within the first few months of life.

376. **(D)** The etiology for secondary amenorrhea is pregnancy, pituitary tumor, menopause, too little body fat, excessive exercise, rapid weight loss, thyroid disease, polycystic ovaries, anorexia or other eating disorders, premature ovarian failure, or Asherman's syndrome (Hawkins et al., 1993).

377. **(A)** When conducting a physical examination on a patient with amenorrhea, the following should be included: patient's height and weight; assessment of the thyroid gland; breast assessment for size and the nipples for discharge (milk, clear, dark, light, bloody, thick or thin); a vaginal examination; and a bimanual examination (Hawkins et al., 1993).

378. **(D)** When a patient presents with amenorrhea, a pregnancy test should always be performed. Approximately 10–20% of amenorrhea is due to hyperprolactinemia (Frederickson & Wilkins-Haug, 1991). Thyroid function tests, including follicle-stimulating hormone (FSH) and luteinizing hormone (LH), will help to identify thyroid disease that may be causing amenorrhea, such as anovulation, Cushing's disease, Addison's disease, and deficiency of dehydroepiandrosterone sulfate. If the patient presents with hirsutism, a testosterone level should be drawn (Emans & Goldstein, 1990; Hawkins et al., 1993).

379. **(D)** If the patient's hCG and prolactin levels are normal, prescribing Provera 10 mg qd for 5 days is the first line of treatment (Hawkins et al., 1993). The next course of action is dependent on the patient's response to the Provera challenge and whether or not the patient is interested in starting on oral contraceptives.

380. **(D)** Primary herpes outbreaks have different clinical symptoms than those that recur. Primary episodes result in local and systemic symptoms, lasting up to 3 weeks on average. More than half of women with a primary infection report fever, headache, malaise, and myalgias. Complaints of dysuria, along with urinary retention and tender inguinal lymphadenopathy, are common complaints (Lichtman & Papera, 1990). While many women with chlamydia remain asymptomatic (50–70%), it is estimated that chlamydia is the number one sexually transmitted disease in Western industrialized societies. Many women present with dysuria and frequency (Star et al., 1995).

381. **(A)** The differential diagnosis for a genital lesion is herpes simplex virus (HSV), syphilis, chancroid, granuloma inguinale, and human papilloma virus (HPV). Urinary tract infections, chlamydia, and gonorrhea are not the differential diagnosis for a genital lesion. Herpes simplex virus (HSV) is transmitted by two types of herpes virus: HSV-I is responsible for oral lesions and lesions above the waist and HSV-II causes infections below the waist. HSV is the most common of vulvar ulcers. Patients present with multiple painful lesions (papules, vesicles, pustules, ulcers, or fissures). Many patients report itching, burning, and/or tingling at the site of the infection and complain of flu-like systemic symptoms

(Star et al., 1995). Syphilis is caused by the motile spirochete *Treponema pallidum.* Patients are often asymptomatic and present with a painless raised lesion. Those presenting with secondary syphilis may have flu-like symptoms (Star et al., 1995). Chancroid is caused by the gram-negative bacillus *Haemophilus ducreyi.*

Cases are rare in the United States, with approximately 5000 cases reported in 1987. These cases are predominantly seen in prostitutes. Symptoms may include external dysuria, painful ulcer, pain on defecation, and rectal bleeding (Star et al., 1995). Lastly, granuloma inguinale is an extremely rare disease in the United States that is caused by a gram-negative bacterium known as *Calymmatobacterium granulomatis,* also called Donovan's body. This infectious agent is believed to be transmitted both sexually and nonsexually. Patients may complain of pruritis and a painless lump in the genital area (Star et al., 1995). Human papilloma virus causes genital warts known as condyloma acuminata. The lesions are usually painless, soft, flat, and flesh-colored and they can appear singularly or in groups (Gerchufsky, 1996).

382.   (D) A provider should never force a patient to have a speculum exam nor should patients be coerced into an exam. Given the patient's history of routinely keeping appointments, and her request not to have a pelvic exam today, obtaining virology cultures of the lesions and an RPR and starting treatment for a case of presumed HSV is reasonable. Obtaining a urine culture to assure that the patient does not have a concomitant infection is also prudent. The patient should return in 3–4 days for follow-up (Star et al, 1995; Hawkins et al., 1993; Lichtman & Papera, 1990).

383.   (C) The correct treatment dose for a patient with a primary outbreak of HSV is acyclovir 200 mg po, 5 times/day for 4–7 days or until clinical resolution is attained. Acyclovir will not cover *Escherichia coli,* and thus treatment with a broad-spectrum sulfa drug is indicated (Ricchini, 1997; Star et al., 1995).

Dermatologic

CASES AND QUESTIONS

Questions 384–388

A 12-year-old, previously healthy child, presents with a 1-day history of pruritic skin lesions. Physical exam reveals circular, elevated lesions with pink edges and central pallor. The lesions appear well circumscribed and range in size from 3 to 8 cm. His history is unremarkable and physical exam is noncontributory, except for the rash.

384. What are the primary characteristics of acute urticaria?

    (A) There are wheals that resolve or change shape within 12 hours.
    (B) There is cutaneous tenderness.
    (C) The face, groin, and neck are most often affected.
    (D) The lesions, when coalesced, do not blanch on pressure.

385. Differential diagnoses to consider in a patient with urticaria include

    (A) Rubeola
    (B) Tinea corporis
    (C) Erythema multiforme
    (D) Erythema infectiosum

386. In food-induced urticaria of infants and young children, the most common offending agents are

    (A) Egg whites, peanuts, and milk
    (B) Food additives, such as red dye

    (C) Sugar
    (D) Tomatoes and citrus fruits

387. Management of the child with urticaria includes

    (A) Systemic corticosteroids when antihistamines are ineffective
    (B) Oral diphenhydramine (5 mg/kg/day)
    (C) Identification and elimination of the causal agent
    (D) All of the above

388. Most cases of drug-induced hives are due to

    (A) Immediate IgA reactions
    (B) Immediate IgE reactions
    (C) Delayed IgG reactions
    (D) Cell-mediated reactions

Questions 389–392

An 8-month-old is evaluated for a worsening diaper rash. Mother reports using corn starch in the diaper area, but the rash has spread from the diaper area to the inner thighs. Physical exam reveals a shiny, confluent, erythematous rash on the convex area of the buttocks and genitalia with sparing of the intertriginous creases. The remainder of the exam was normal.

389. Which of the following is the most common cause of diaper dermatitis?

    (A) Impetigo
    (B) Atopic dermatitis
    (C) Psoriasis
    (D) Irritant contact dermatitis

390. What are the features of the candidiasis rash that distinguishes it from irritant diaper dermatitis?

(A) The lesions appear bright, beefy red with sharp, raised borders.
(B) The rash has a characteristic salmon-colored greasy appearance with yellow scale.
(C) The lesions appear glistening and erythematous and spare the creases.
(D) The rash presents as bullae, 1–2 cm in diameter, with regional lymphadenopathy.

391. What is the preferred treatment for diaper dermatitis due to *Candida albicans?*

(A) Topical high-potency corticosteroids
(B) Topical antibiotic mupirocin cream
(C) Topical antifungals, such as nystatin or clotrimazole
(D) Moisture-resistant barrier ointments

392. Characteristics of oral candidiasis (thrush) include which of the following?

(A) Mild fever, arthralgia, and macular-papular eruptions
(B) Adherent creamy white plaques with mucosal ulceration
(C) Grouped vesicles, fever, and diarrhea
(D) Palatal petechiae, dysphagia, and local lymphadenopathy

Questions 393–396

A 3-year-old presents with a group of lesions that began as presumptive insect bites on the child's lower left leg. These lesions have advanced from papules to vesicopustules to a honey-crusted area on an erythematous base. The physical exam is noncontributory, except for a few enlarged, nontender, left inguinal lymph nodes. The child is afebrile.

393. The most likely cause of this child's current lesions is

(A) Flea bite hypersensitivity
(B) Herpes simplex
(C) Tinea corporis
(D) Impetigo

394. Which of the following organisms are most commonly responsible for superficial bacterial infections of the epidermis?

(A) *Staphylococcs aureus* and group A beta hemolytic streptococci
(B) Group A beta hemolytic streptococci and *Haemophilus influenza* type B
(C) *Haemophilus influenza* type B and group B streptococci
(D) *Streptococcus pneumoniae* and herpes simplex

395. What is the recommended treatment of most localized, superficial, bacterial infections of the epidermis?

(A) Topical therapy with antimicrobials
(B) Oral therapy with sulfonamides
(C) Vigorous cleaning of the affected area only
(D) None of the above

396. Which of the following is a *true* statement concerning bacterial infections of the skin?

(A) Cellulitis should be treated only in children with fever or systemic symptoms.
(B) Bullous impetigo is caused by an epidermolytic toxin-producing strain of *S. aureus.*
(C) The rash of scarlet fever is characterized by papulovesicular eruptions in the flexor folds.
(D) Bacterial infections of the skin are generally resistant to penicillin-derivative therapy.

Questions 397–402

Helen is a 4-year-old brought in by her mother for an itchy rash that has appeared over the past 2 weeks in the intragluteal area of her groin and the webs of her fingers. She seems to be most pruritic at night. She has been afebrile, is on no medications, and has had no associated symptoms. Other family members have had similar symptoms. On exam, she is found to have tiny, excoriated papules and evidence of a linear burrow on her finger web. Her physical exam is normal except for her skin findings.

397. Based on the history and physical exam, what is the most likely reason for this child's rash?

(A) Atopic dermatitis
(B) Candidiasis
(C) Scabies
(D) Seborrheic dermatitis

398. A linear burrow on the skin can be best described as

(A) A tunnel in which a female mite deposits eggs from which larvae emerge
(B) A hypersensitivity reaction to an arthropod bite
(C) A cell-mediated response
(D) None of the above

399. Effective scabicide therapy in older children includes

(A) Permethrin 5% cream
(B) Crotamiton
(C) Lindane
(D) All of the above

400. Which of the following topical scabicides is *not* recommended for use in young children?

(A) Pyrethrins (RID, A-200 Pyrinate)
(B) Crotamiton (Eurax)
(C) Permethrin (Nix, Elimite)
(D) Lindane (Kwell)

401. Which of the following body sites are *not* commonly affected in adolescents and older persons with scabies?

(A) Finger webs and sides of the digits
(B) Head, neck, palms, and soles of the feet
(C) Fingers, axillae, and waistline
(D) Umbilicus, groin, and genital region

402. Differential diagnoses of pruritic lesions of the scalp include

(A) Nummular eczema
(B) Alopecia areata
(C) Pediculosis capitis
(D) Caput succedaneum

Questions 403–407

A 5-month-old boy, Jedidiah, presents for his well-child visit. His mother states that he has had an erythematous, confluent, and scaly rash on his face and on the extensor surfaces of his extremities for the past month. She has treated it with baby oil and tar soap. He is receiving no medication except for Dimetapp on occasion for rhinorrhea. His history is significant for one wheezing episode in the past month and an allergy to cow's milk. His family history is positive for asthma and hay fever. Vital signs are normal and his physical exam is normal except for the presence of the rash.

403. The most likely diagnosis for this child's rash is

(A) Tinea corporis
(B) Atopic dermatitis
(C) Psoriasis
(D) Viral exanthem

404. Which of the following statements is *not* true regarding the rash of atopic dermatitis?

(A) The rash of the older child is usually not pruritic.
(B) Excessive skin dryness is a concomitant finding.
(C) Scratching may predispose the patient to skin infection.
(D) In infancy there is often facial and extensor involvement.

405. Appropriate management of this child's condition includes

(A) Topical steroids and reduction of dryness and irritation
(B) Topical antifungals
(C) Oral antimicrobials and good hygiene
(D) Moisture-resistant barrier ointment or cream

406. The diagnosis of atopic disease can be aided by which of the following laboratory findings?

    (A) Elevated serum IgE concentrations
    (B) Skin scrapings
    (C) Elevated serum antinuclear antibody (ANA)
    (D) None of the above

407. Of the following statements, which best represents the prognosis of atopic dermatitis?

    (A) There is a high likelihood that the child with atopic dermatitis will develop allergic rhinitis or asthma.
    (B) Avoidance of an identified food may prove beneficial in controlling symptoms.
    (C) Breast-feeding may delay the onset of atopic dermatitis.
    (D) All of the above.

Questions 408–411

A 5-year-old, Elias, is evaluated for a 2-day history of fever with a temperature of 39.2°C (102.6°F), runny nose, decreased appetite, and a rash on his trunk. He is in kindergarten and he has had no ill contacts. He is on no current medications except for acetaminophen for fever. He has no history of dermatologic problems. On physical exam, his vital signs are stable with a temperature of 38°C (100.4°F). orally. His appearance is nontoxic. The exam is normal except for scattered, erythematous, macular-papular, and vesicular lesions on his trunk.

408. What is the most likely cause of this exanthem?

    (A) Scabies
    (B) Arthropod (tick) bite
    (C) Scarletina
    (D) Varicella

409. Key points in the history of a patient with an exanthem include which of the following?

    (A) Has the child had any infectious contacts?
    (B) Does the child have a history of similar lesions?

    (C) Does the child have any associated symptoms such as fever, runny nose, or cough?
    (D) All of the above

410. Treatment of a child with uncomplicated varicella includes

    (A) Topical diphenhydramine
    (B) Nonaspirin antipyretics
    (C) Varicella-zoster immune globulin (VZIG)
    (D) Systemic acyclovir therapy

411. *True* statements concerning herpes zoster (shingles) include

    (A) Patients with zoster can transmit the virus to susceptible contacts, who will develop primary varicella.
    (B) The incidence of reactivation of the varicella virus decreases with age.
    (C) The treatment of zoster infection includes intramuscular VZIG injection.
    (D) The rash of zoster consists of widespread vesicular lesions on the trunk and extremities.

Questions 412–415

A 14-year-old male comes in to a school-based health center to be seen for a sports physical. His exam is unremarkable, except for some mild inflammatory acne on his forehead, chin, and back.

412. Which of the following factors has *not* been found to contribute to the development of acne eruptions?

    (A) Intake of foods such as chocolate, soda, and french fries
    (B) Genetic and hormonal factors
    (C) Specific drugs such as oral contraceptive pills (OCP)
    (D) External agents such as skin bacteria

413. The pathogenesis of the primary lesion of acne is best described as

    (A) Infection of the sebaceous gland
    (B) An immunologic response to bacteria

(C) Plugging of the sebaceous gland

(D) Inflammation deep within the dermal layer

414. Initial treatment of the adolescent with mild to moderate acne includes

(A) Oral isotretinoin (Accutane)

(B) Topical tretinoin (Retin-A) and benzoyl peroxide gel

(C) Systemic antibiotics such as tetracycline

(D) Vigorous scrubbing with a non-abrasive soap only

415. Which of the following factors is *least* likely to be related to the severity of acne?

(A) Increased stress

(B) Poor hygiene

(C) Increased sebum production

(D) Age of the patient

Questions 416–418

A 3-week-old male presents with a scaly rash on the scalp and some scaling behind the ears. The infant's mother has been bathing him regularly, using baby shampoo on his scalp. The infant has been otherwise well. He received the hepatitis B vaccine at birth. His family history is significant for Lyme disease in the infant's father. The infant's weight is 30th percentile. His vital signs are normal and his physical exam is normal except for the presence of a rash.

416. Which of the following is the most likely diagnosis of this infant's rash?

(A) Irritant contact dermatitis

(B) Tinea capitis

(C) Alopecia areata

(D) Seborrheic dermatitis

417. Initial management of this disorder includes

(A) Oral antibiotic therapy

(B) Shampoos containing sulfur or salicylic acid

(C) Topical antifungal medication

(D) All of the above

418. Which of the following is *not* a true statement concerning these dermatologic disorders?

(A) Seborrheic dermatitis occurs predominantly in infancy and puberty.

(B) Seborrheic dermatitis can be distinguished from atopic dermatitis by a lack of significant pruritis.

(C) Psoriasis is a common papulosquamous eruption that is presumed to be viral in origin.

(D) Alopecia areata is the most common cause of hair loss in children.

Questions 419–422

Rebekah, an 8-year-old, presents for evaluation of multiple warts on her fingers and hands. Her history and physical exam are noncontributory, except for persistent nail biting. A diagnosis of verruca vulgaris (common warts) is made.

419. Common warts are caused by which of the following viruses?

(A) Ebstein-Barr virus (EBV)

(B) Pox virus

(C) Herpes simplex virus type I

(D) Human papilloma virus types 1, 2, 4, and 7

420. Which of the following statements is *true* concerning anogenital warts in children?

(A) Anogenital warts can occur from non-sexual contact with infected caretakers.

(B) Podophyllin is the treatment of choice in genital warts.

(C) Perinatal contact through an infected birth canal is a common source of infection in infants.

(D) All of the above.

421. Which of the following conditions puts a child at high risk for developing warts?

(A) Long-term use of antibiotic therapy

(B) Immunodeficiency

(C) Insulin-dependent diabetes mellitus

(D) None of the above

422. Superficial pearly papules with umbilicated centers best describes which of the following skin disorders?

    (A) Molluscum contagiosum
    (B) Xanthomas
    (C) Verruca vulgaris
    (D) Herpes zoster

Questions 423–428

A 10-year-old is brought in for a pruritic rash on the thigh and trunk. She is otherwise well, except for a recent mild viral illness. Her immunization status is up to date and no family members are ill at this time. She has received no medications and has no allergies. Physical exam reveals an oval plaque with central clearing and a scaly border on her right thigh. Smaller papular lesions are evident on the trunk. Her exam is otherwise normal.

423. What is the most likely diagnosis of this child's disorder?

    (A) Henoch-Schönlein purpura (HSP)
    (B) Pityriasis rosea
    (C) Scabies
    (D) Erythema multiforme (EM)

424. All the following rash characteristics are associated with this disorder EXCEPT

    (A) Herald patch
    (B) Christmas tree pattern
    (C) Mild pruritis
    (D) Areas of depigmentation

425. What is the natural history of this rash?

    (A) Resolves in 4–12 weeks without treatment
    (B) Resolves in 4–6 months without treatment
    (C) Resolves in 4–6 months with systemic antiviral therapy
    (D) Resolves in 9–12 months with systemic corticosteroids

426. A common fungal infection of the skin that produces red, scaly, round lesions is

    (A) Herpes simplex
    (B) Tinea corporis
    (C) Pityriasis alba
    (D) Vitiligo

427. What test confirms the diagnosis of this fungal dermatosis?

    (A) Tzanck smear of the lesion
    (B) Serum erythrocyte sedimentation rate (ESR)
    (C) Potassium hydroxide (KOH) exam of the skin
    (D) Serum IgE

428. Recommended treatment in mild cases of this fungal dermatosis is

    (A) Topical imidazole cream
    (B) Topical corticosteroids
    (C) Topical antihistamine
    (D) Permethrin cream 5%

ANSWERS AND RATIONALES

384. **(A)** An urticarial rash is acute in onset, evanescent, and intensely pruritic. It appears as raised, erythematous lesions of various sizes, with pale centers and pink borders. They become scattered or more generalized, may become confluent, may blanch on pressure, and are not generally painful.

385. **(C)** Erythema multiforme (EM) is a cutaneous disorder that is believed to represent an immune complex reaction. The most common etiologic factors are medications and infections. Erythema multiforme has an abrupt onset, is characterized by a variety of lesions, favors the extremities, including palms and soles, and ranges in severity from mild to severe disease (Stevens-Johnson syndrome) (Frieden, 1996). (See Table A385, p. 138.)

386. **(A)** Foods are the most common types of allergens to cause acute urticaria. After ingesting the offending food, lesions may appear around the mouth and may cause the oropharynx to swell. The most common offending agents in infants and young children are egg whites, peanuts, and milk, with peanuts, fish, and shellfish the most common offending agents in older children. Strawberries, citrus, and tomatoes may cause hives, but are not the most common offending agents (Buckley, 1996).

387. **(D)** The main goal of therapy in acute urticaria is to relieve itching, burning, and swelling. Antihistamines, such as diphenhydramine (Benadryl), are useful. If combinations of antihistamines do not prove effective, oral steroids can be used in a tapered regimen (Schiff, 1996). Most importantly, the offending agent should be identified through a careful, detailed history.

388. **(B)** Acute urticaria is due to type I, IgE-mediated immunologic reactions. They tend to cause symptoms within hours after exposure and are rarely the cause of chronic hives (> 6–8 weeks). Histamine may be released as a consequence of IgE antigen–antibody reactions.

389. **(D)** Irritant contact dermatitis is a common dermatologic problem in young children. It is caused by prolonged contact of the skin with urine and feces, which contain irritating chemicals. In 80% of cases of diaper dermatitis lasting > 3 days, the affected area has become colonized with *Candida albicans* (Morelli & Weston, 1997).

390. **(A)** *Candida albicans* can be a source of diaper dermatitis or can cause a secondary infection on already inflamed skin. The rash appears bright, beefy red with sharp, raised borders and satellite papules, vesicles, and pustules along the margins. It can be distinguished from irritant contact dermatitis by the distribution of the lesions to the intertriginous folds. Although the diagnosis of candidiasis is usually made on clinical grounds, a skin scraping with KOH may be performed that would demonstrate budding yeast with hyphae and pseudohyphae (Weinberg & Levin, 1997).

391. **(C)** Management of irritant diaper dermatitis usually responds to hygienic measures, the application of barrier ointments, and a low-potency topical hydrocortisone cream. Candidal diaper dermatitis is best treated by topical antifungal creams, such as nystatin, miconazole, or clotrimazole, in addition to a topical, mild corticosteroid cream, such as hydrocortisone 1% (Weinberg & Levin, 1997).

392. **(B)** The organism *Candida albicans,* which causes candidal diaper dermatits, is also responsible for oral candidiasis (thrush). Thrush is very common in otherwise healthy infants. Oral candidiasis is characterized by adherent, white plaques that often resemble formula, but cannot be removed with a tongue blade or swab. These lesions can be found on the buccal mucosa, palate, and tongue. Recommended treatment is with oral nystatin 100,000 units 4–6 times a day until resolution (Weinberg & Levin, 1997). Eradication of candida from pacifiers, bottle nipples, toys, or mother's breasts may be helpful as well.

393. **(D)** Impetigo is a very common bacterial skin infection in children. Predisposing factors are warm weather, localized areas of skin trauma, and preexisting skin disorders, such as atopic dermatitis (Frieden, 1996). The face, arms, and legs are most commonly affected. The affected child is often systemically well, although he or she may have localized lymphadenopathy.

394. **(A)** The predominant organisms implicated in impetigo are *S. aureus* or group A beta-hemolytic streptococcus, or a combination of both organisms.

395. **(A)** The treatment of choice for impetigo is that which has coverage for staphylococcal organisms. In localized infection, topical antibiotics such as bacitracin, polymyxin B, or mupirocin can be used. In the case of widespread lesions, oral treatment, such as dicloxicillin, cephalexin, amoxicillin–clavulanate, and erythromycin, is recommended. In light of the data concerning staph resistance to erythromycin, providers should select antibiotic coverage based on the current resistance patterns in their communities.

396. **(B)** Bullous impetigo is one of the dermatologic manifestations of a toxin-producing

strain of *Staphylococcus aureus.* The diagnosis can be made by obtaining a Gram's stain of the denuded skin or bullous fluid. The classic lesions are bullae filled with cloudy fluid that are surrounded by a thin area of erythema. These lesions are very contagious and parenteral treatment is usually indicated.

397. **(C)** Scabies is a common infestation caused by *Sarcoptes scabiei.* It is highly contagious and is characterized by papular eruptions that are very pruritic. These erythematous papules may become excoriated and secondarily infected.

398. **(A)** A superficial, gray, threadlike line in the skin is a result of the adult female scabies mite burrowing into the skin to deposit eggs. Within 10 days, these pass through the larval and nymphal stages to become adults. Their life span is about 1 month. Skin scrapings of the burrow can be examined by microscopy to identify the scabies mite in an affected individual. Sixty percent of patients who are symptomatic can be found to have mites, eggs, and/or feces of the mite (Frieden, 1996).

399. **(D)** Several topical scabicides are available for the treatment of scabies. This therapy should be used for all members of the household as well as all close contacts (ie, sexual). The three medications that are used to treat scabies in the older child are lindane 1% (Kwell), crotamiton 10% (Eurax), and permethrin (Elimite) as a single application. Additional medications that may play a role in scabies therapy include antihistamines, such as hydroxyzine to reduce pruritis, and a mild topical steroid to decrease the inflammatory response to the mite (Berkowitz, 1996).

400. **(D)** In light of the concern over absorption of lindane (Kwell) and its potential neurotoxicity, its use is not recommended in infants, young children, or pregnant or breast-feeding women. Alternative medications, such as permethrin 5% cream (Elimite), are the treatment of choice in these circumstances (Morelli & Weston, 1997).

401. **(B)** In infants and in young children, scabetic lesions are often found on the scalp, neck, palms, and soles of the feet. In contrast, preferred body sites in older children are the finger webs, axillae, nipples, groin, and intragluteal area.

402. **(C)** Pediculosis capitis (head lice) is a very common childhood infestation caused by the louse, *Pediculus capitis.* School-age children are most frequently infected, particularly girls. Infestations can occur from close contacts or from fomites. Children who are infected often present with intense scalp itch or visible nits or lice in the scalp (Honig, 1986).

403. **(B)** Atopic dermatitis is a common skin disorder that frequently occurs in infancy and is chronic in nature. It is characterized by erythema and papulovesicular and exudative inflammation. There is a strong association between atopic dermatitis and allergic rhinitis and asthma. Two-thirds to three-quarters of children with this disorder have a positive family history of atopic disease (Cohen, 1992). The exact cause is unknown; however, it is thought to have an immunologic basis.

404. **(A)** The rash of atopic dermatitis is characterized by marked pruritis and by acute and chronic changes in the skin. The age of the child determines the patterns of presentation. In the infantile form, the face and extensor surfaces are commonly affected, with the diaper area spared. In the older child, the flexural areas are more involved and the face spared. Associated findings include dryness and tendency toward skin infections, such as bacterial infections, herpes simplex, and molluscum contagiosum (Williams, 1996).

405. **(A)** Treatment goals of atopic dermatitis are principally to reduce itching, lubricate the skin with emollient creams, and reduce inflammation through the use of topical corticosteroids. Other medications, such as antimicrobials, are reserved for the treatment of superinfections of the skin.

406. **(A)** For most patients, the diagnosis of atopic dermatitis can be made through clinical findings and elevated serum IgE concentrations. Atopic children will frequently have positive skin tests to foods such as egg whites, peanuts, cow's milk, wheat, and soybean (Williams, 1996). Ingestion of these foods can provoke exacerbation of the symptoms in the atopic child. In infancy, avoiding allergens, prolonging breast-feeding, and delaying the introduction of solids may delay the onset of atopic dermatitis but will not prevent its development in the future (Halbert, 1996).

407. **(D)** There is no complete cure for atopic disease. Although many cases resolve spontaneously in childhood, the more severe cases can lead to persistent symptoms into adolescence and adulthood. Between 50 and 80% of children with eczema may go on to develop either allergic rhinitis, asthma, or both (Williams, 1996). If a food allergen is found to be causative, eliminating it may be beneficial. Breast-feeding may delay but not eliminate the onset of eczema (Heyman et al., 1997).

408. **(D)** Varicella (chicken pox) is a common childhood exanthem caused by the varicella-zoster virus. It has a higher incidence in late winter and early spring, is highly contagious, and is spread by respiratory droplets to susceptible individuals. The lesions begin as small papules and progress to vesicles on an erythematous base, which ulcerates and becomes a small scab.

409. **(D)** A thorough history should be obtained in a child with an exanthem. Additional questions to ask in order to aid in diagnosis include the child's immunization status, any medication use, and a recent travel history.

410. **(B)** Treatment of varicella is directed toward relieving discomfort from symptoms such as fever and itching. Fever can be treated with acetaminophen or ibuprofen. Aspirin products should be avoided because of their association with Reye's syndrome, a serious disease that involves liver dysfunction and encephalopathy (AAP, 1997).

411. **(A)** Zoster is the reactivation of the varicella-zoster virus that has been dormant after clinical chicken pox (Pattishall, 1997). Children who have had varicella early in life (before 1 year of age) have an increased incidence of zoster later in life. Zoster infections can lead to primary varicella in exposure to susceptible individuals.

412. **(A)** Acne vulgaris is a common condition that affects 95% and 83% of 16-year-old boys and girls, respectively (Healy & Simpson, 1994). It is a multifactorial disease and several factors are thought to contribute to its development. These include endogenous hormones, some drugs, some external agents such as skin bacteria, industrial chemicals, and oil- or wax-containing cosmetics. Foods such as caffeinated drinks, chocolate, and fried foods have not been shown to cause or worsen acne (Sifuentes, 1996).

413. **(C)** The initial pathogenesis of the acne lesion is the development of comedones, which are small cysts that contain debris that is formed by plugging of the sebaceous gland (Prose, 1996).

414. **(B)** The adolescent with mild to moderate acne would benefit from topical tretinoin to prevent comedone formation and benzoyl peroxide gel, which has both antibacterial and comedolytic activities. Oral retinoids are known to be teratogenic to a fetus in the first trimester of pregnancy, and oral antibiotics are used in patients who do not respond to topical therapy. Patients with acne should practice good hygiene; however, excessive scrubbing is not recommended.

415. **(B)** Acne vulgaris is a disorder of adolescence. The severity of acne can be affected by sebum production, which is the secretory product of the sebaceous gland. The reason behind the worsening of acne during stress is unclear (Hurwitz, 1994). Excessive scrubbing with abrasive soaps is not found to be effective in preventing new lesions. Inflammation of the skin surface can occur when comedones are traumatized by the patient.

416. **(D)** Seborrheic dermatitis is a common dermatosis that often develops during the first 3 months of life and may be influenced by androgenic hormones (Herbert & Goller, 1996). It is characterized by scaliness on the scalp, behind the ears, and in the intertriginous areas. It occurs primarily in infancy and puberty and can be distinguished from atopic dermatitis by a lack of significant pruritis (Pearlman, Greos, & Vitanza, 1997).

417. **(B)** Seborrheic dermatitis can easily be treated by the use of a shampoo containing mild salicylic acid or sulfur. Shampoo should be left on the scalp for 10 minutes and the eye area should be avoided (Hebert & Goller, 1996). Co-infections with candida may occur and can be treated with antifungals such as clotrimazole, whereas secondary infection with bacteria would necessitate treatment with antibiotics.

418. **(C)** Psoriasis is a chronic papulosquamous eruption characterized by erythematous papules covered by thick, white scales. Lesions can occur anywhere on the body, but more commonly occur on the elbows, knees, and scalp. Psoriasis has no known cause, but is thought to have a polygenic inheritance pattern (Hebert & Goller, 1996). It requires a series of medications, although topical steroids are a mainstay of therapy.

419. **(D)** Verruca vulgaris (common warts) are benign epidermal tumors that are produced from human papilloma virus (HPV) types 1, 2, 4, and 7 infection of the skin. They are commonly seen on the fingers, hands, and feet. Local trauma contributes to inoculation of the virus (Cohen, 1993).

420. **(D)** Anogenital warts are a common complaint in sexually active adolescents as well as in prepubertal children. Although children may acquire anogenital warts through nonsexual contact with caretakers, through sib-

lings who have genital HPV or common warts, or through an infected birth canal, the possibility of sexual abuse should be investigated (Cohen, 1997).

421. **(B)** Although warts are often a persistent and frustrating problem, most warts will spontaneously resolve without treatment in healthy individuals. Immunocompromised hosts, however, are susceptible to developing widespread lesions that may produce functional impairment and psychosocial consequences (Cohen, 1997).

422. **(A)** Molluscum contagiosum is a cutaneous viral infection caused by the large pox virus. It is characterized by dome-shaped papules that are superficial, pearly colored, and with umbilicated centers. Lesions are often found on the trunk, axillae, face, and diaper area and are spread by scratching. Most lesions resolve without treatment; however, widespread lesions should be referred to a dermatologist and the individual should be evaluated for immunodeficiency disease (Cohen, 1993).

423. **(B)** Pityriasis rosea is a self-limiting disorder common in school-age children and young adults. Peak incidence is in late winter and the cause is unknown. A prodrome of malaise, headache, and constitutional symptoms may precede the rash (Cohen, 1993).

424. **(D)** The rash of pityriasis rosea is characterized by an eruption that is known as a herald patch,

which is oval shaped, pink, and scaly. Over 1–2 weeks, many lesions can appear on the body that run parallel to the skin lines of the thorax and back, creating a "Christmas tree" pattern. This rash can be mildly pruritic, and in dark-skinned individuals, post-inflammation hyperpigmentation may occur (Cohen, 1993).

425. **(A)** Most patients with pityriasis rosea require no treatment, with the rash slowly fading over 4–12 weeks. Mild pruritis can be managed with oral antihistamines. In more severe cases, ultraviolet light (UVB) may be used to hasten the disappearance of the rash (Prose, 1996).

426. **(B)** Tinea corporis (ringworm) is a common skin disorder in children and is primarily caused by the organism *Trichophyton tonsurans*. The characteristic lesion is that of pruritic annular plaques with central clearing or scale, and with an erythematous border. It is acquired from direct human contact or from an infected domestic animal (Frieden, 1996).

427. **(C)** The diagnosis of tinea corporis can be confirmed through examination of a scraping of the skin lesion treated with 20% KOH solution. Evidence of fungal hyphae on a KOH prep is considered diagnostic of tinea corporis (Frieden, 1996).

428. **(A)** The treatment of mild tinea corporis can be accomplished through the use of topical antifungal creams (imidazoles). If the infection is extensive, oral griseofulvin or ketoconazole may be necessary (Frieden, 1996).

TABLE A385. RED RASHES IN CHILDREN

Condition	Incubation Period (Days)	Prodrome	Rash	Laboratory Tests	Comments, Other Diagnostic Features
Measles	9–14	Cough, rhinitis, conjunctivitis	Maculopapular, face to extremities; lasts 7–10 d; Koplik's spots in mouth	Leukopenia	Toxic. Bright red rash becomes confluent, may desquamate.
Rubella	14–21	Usually none	Mild maculopapular; rapid spread face to extremities; gone by day 4	Normal or leukopenia	Postauricular, occipital adenopathy common. Polyarthralgia in some older girls. Mild clinical illness.
Roseola (exanthem subitum)	10–14	Fever (3–4 d)	Pink, macular rash occurs at end of illness; transient	Normal	Fever often high, and disappears when rash develops; child appears well. Usually occurs in children 6 m–2 y of age.
Erythema infectiosum	13–18	None	Erythematous "slapped" cheeks; then reticular rash on extremities, trunk	Normal (reticulocytopenia)	Rash may reappear over weeks, especially with exposure to heat, sunlight. May cause arthralgia/arthritis, usually in older children or adults. Red cell maturation arrest in children with chronic hemolysis can cause aplastic crisis.
Enterovirus	2–7	Variable fever, chills, myalgia, sore throat	Usually macular, maculopapular on trunk or palms, soles; vesicles, petechiae also seen	Variable	Varied rashes may resemble those of many other infections. Pharyngeal or hand-foot-mouth vesicles may occur.
Streptococcal scarlet fever	1–7	Fever, abdominal pain, headache, sore throat	Diffuse erythema, "sandpaper" texture; neck, axillae, inguinal areas; spreads to rest of body; desquamates 7–14 d	Leukocytosis; positive group A streptococcus culture of throat or wound	Strawberry tongue, red pharynx with or without exudate. Eyes, perioral and periorbital area, palms, and soles spared. Pastia's lines. Brief prodrome. Cervical adenopathy, mild, variant, scarlatina. Usually occurs in children 2–10 y of age.
Staphylococcal scarlet fever	1–7	Variable fever	Diffuse erythroderma; resembles streptococcal scarlet fever except eyes may be hyperemic, no "strawberry" tongue, pharynx spared	Variable leukocytosis if infected	Focal *Staphylococcus aureus* infection usually present.
Staphylococcal scalded skin	Variable	Irritability, absent to low fever	Painful erythroderma, followed in 1–2 d by dry cracking around eyes, mouth; bullae form with friction (Nikolsky's sign)	Normal if only colonized by staph; leukocytosis and sometimes bacteremia if infected	Normal pharynx. Look for focal staph infection. Usually occurs in infants.
Toxic shock syndrome	Variable	Fever, myalgia, headache, diarrhea, vomiting	Nontender erythroderma; red eyes, palms, soles, pharynx, lips	Leukocytosis; abnormal liver enzymes, coagulation tests; proteinuria	*S. aureus* infection, multiorgan involvement. Swollen hands, feet. Hypotension or shock.
Erythema multiforme	—	Usually none or related to underlying cause	Discrete, red maculopapular lesions; symmetric, distal, palms and soles; target lesions classic	Normal or eosinophilia	Reaction to drugs (especially sulfas), or infectious agents. Urticaria, arthralgia also seen.

(continued)

TABLE A385. *(Continued)*

Condition	Incubation Period (Days)	Prodrome	Rash	Laboratory Tests	Comments, Other Diagnostic Features
Stevens-Johnson syndrome	—	Pharyngitis, conjunctivitis, fever, malaise	Bullous erythema multiforme; may slough in large areas; hemorrhagic lips; purulent conjunctivitis	Leukocytosis	Classic precipitants are drugs (especially sulfas), *Mycoplasma pneumoniae* and herpes simplex infections. Pneumonitis and urethritis also seen.
Drug allergy	—	None, fever alone, or fever, myalgia, pruritus	Macular, maculopapular, urticarial, or erythroderma	Leukopenia, eosinophila	Rash variable. Severe reactions may resemble measles, scarlet fever; adenopathy, hepatosplenomegaly, marked toxicity possible.
Kawasaki disease	Unknown	Fever, cervical adenopathy, irritability	Polymorphous (may be erythroderma) on trunk and extremities; red palms and soles, lips, tongue, pharynx	Leukocytosis, thrombocytosis, elevated ESR; pyuria; negative cultures and streptococcal serology	Swollen hands, feet; prolonged illness; bulbar hyperemia; uveitis; aseptic meningitis; no response to antibiotics. Vasculitis and aneurysms of coronary and other arteries occur.
Leptospirosis	4–19	Fever, myalgia, chills	Variable erythroderma	Leukocytosis; hematuria, proteinuria; hyperbilirubinema	Conjunctivitis; toxic. Hepatitis, aseptic meningitis may be seen. Rodent, dog contact.

Reprinted with permission from Levin, M.J. (1997). Infections: Viral & rickettsial. In W.W. Hay, J.R. Groothuis, A.R. Hayward, & M.J. Levin, eds. Current pediatric diagnosis and treatment (13th ed.). Stamford, CT: Appleton & Lange.

Musculoskeletal

CASES AND QUESTIONS

Questions 429–432

Matthew is a 5-year-old male who presents today with a sudden-onset limp and right hip pain that began earlier today. There is no reported trauma or falls. He attends preschool 3 days/week and has had a URI without fever for 3 days.

429. Differential diagnosis of a painful limp includes all of the following EXCEPT

    (A) Trauma
    (B) Musculoskeletal neoplasms
    (C) Slipped capital femoral epiphysis
    (D) Duchenne's muscular dystrophy

Physical examination reveals a nontoxic child, T 38.4°C (101.2°F), with insignificant abdominal, knee, and HEENT exams. There is limitation of active and passive right hip joint motion with no tenderness or erythema.

430. Which of the following diagnostic tests would be most appropriate to obtain for this patient?

    1. CBC with differential
    2. Hip x-rays
    3. ESR
    4. Aspiration of R hip joint
       (A) 1, 2, and 3
       (B) 1, 2, 3, and 4
       (C) 1 only
       (D) 1, 2, and 4

431. All diagnostic tests show normal values. Imaging studies are entirely normal. The most likely cause of this 5-year-old's limp is

    (A) Trauma
    (B) Transient synovitis
    (C) Septic arthritis
    (D) Legg-Calvé-Perthes disease

432. Appropriate management of this child would include all the following EXCEPT

    (A) Restriction of physical activity and weight bearing
    (B) Analgesic for pain such as ibuprofen or acetaminophen
    (C) Prompt referral to an orthopedist for hospitalization and traction
    (D) Close at-home observation and follow-up in 48 hours

Questions 433–435

Sarah is a 2-week-old, full-term, healthy infant. She presents today for a health supervision visit with her mother and grandmother. Sarah's grandmother expresses concern because "Sarah's foot turns in."

433. The most common congenital foot deformity is

    (A) Metatarsus adductus
    (B) Pes planus
    (C) Eqinovarus
    (D) Femoral anteversion

On physical examination, you can passively correct the forefoot to neutral position. Hip examination is normal bilaterally and there is no torticollis. You suspect supple metatarsus adductus as the cause of this infant's in-toeing.

434. All the following statements regarding supple metatarsus adductus are true EXCEPT

(A) It usually occurs secondary to intrauterine positioning
(B) A majority of infants do not require treatment and have resolution with growth
(C) Corrective shoes are required
(D) Internal tibial torsion is frequently present

435. Appropriate management of this infant would include

(A) Immediate orthopedic referral
(B) No intervention necessary at this time
(C) Serial casting
(D) Forefoot stretching exercises tid

Questions 436–438

Eric is a 22-month-old male who is new to your hospital-based practice. You observe that he has an in-toeing gait.

436. The most common cause of toeing-in in children less than age 2 years is

(A) Genu valgum
(B) Genu varum
(C) Femoral anteversion
(D) Internal tibial torsion

On physical examination, you note that his kneecaps point straight ahead with ambulation, but the feet turn in. Examination of the lower extremities is otherwise unremarkable. There is no falling, limping, or tripping with running or walking.

437. Based on the history and physical examination, you suspect this toddler's in-toeing is most likely due to

(A) Genu valgum
(B) Genu varum
(C) Femoral anteversion
(D) Internal tibial torsion

438. Appropriate management of this toddler would include

(A) Night (Denis Browne) splints
(B) Referral to an orthopedic surgeon
(C) Evaluation at all well-child visits and reassurance that most children have spontaneous correction with growth
(D) Corrective shoes

Questions 439–442

Anita is a 7-hour-old Caucasian female born to a 32-year-old gravida 1, para 1 mother. She was born by elective caesarean section at full term due to breech presentation. Her birth weight is 8 lb 1 oz, with a length of 21 inches. Family and prenatal histories are entirely negative. Upon your initial observation, Anita is noted to be quiet, alert, and moving all extremities symmetrically.

439. Which of the following would most significantly increase Anita's risk of developmental dysplasia of the hip (DDH)?

(A) Elective caesarian section
(B) Breech presentation
(C) Birth weight and length
(D) Gravida 1, para 1 mother

Ortolani and Barlow techniques reveal a "clunk" on the left side and left hip abduction of 50 degrees. Examination of the right hip is entirely normal. While prone, Anita's gluteal skin folds are noted to be asymmetrical.

440. All the following statements regarding DDH are *true* EXCEPT

(A) Routine radiographic studies are helpful in diagnosing DDH in newborns.
(B) DDH is more common in female infants than in male infants.
(C) Diagnosis of DDH in the newborn is made primarily by physical examination.
(D) The etiology of DDH is often multifactorial.

441. Anita is referred to an orthopedist for further evaluation and treatment. The goal of early detection and treatment of DDH is

    (A) To shorten the necessary course of treatment
    (B) To prevent avascular necrosis
    (C) To restore the articulation of the femur within the acetabulum
    (D) All of the above

442. The most likely management of a dislocated hip in a newborn would include

    (A) Observation of the newborn's hip over a three month period
    (B) Traction with surgical reduction
    (C) Pavlik harness to maintain the hip in flexion and abduction
    (D) Triple diapering for 3 months

Questions 443–445

Nick is an 11-year-old male who presents today with a 2-day history of right knee swelling and tenderness. He initially fell off his bicycle and scraped his knee prior to these symptoms. He is unable to fully bear weight on his right leg. He is feeling fatigued today and his temperature at this visit is 39°C (102.2°F). On physical examination he is somewhat toxic-appearing and has limited ROM of his right knee, with diffuse pain to passive movement and palpation over his distal femur. *Laboratory tests:* CBC with differential shows an elevated WBC count and elevated ESR. A blood culture is pending.

443. Based on the this child's health history, physical examination, and diagnostic tests, the most likely diagnosis is

    (A) Osteosarcoma
    (B) Septic arthritis
    (C) Osteomyelitis
    (D) Juvenile rheumatoid arthritis

444. The most common bacterial pathogen causing acute osteomyelitis is

    (A) *Pseudomonas aeruginosa*
    (B) *Staphylococcus aureus*
    (C) Salmonella
    (D) *Haemophilus influenzae*

445. The most appropriate management of this patient would be

    (A) X-ray of R leg and hip and refer to orthopedist
    (B) Immediate orthopedic referral for evaluation, hospitalization, and IV antibiotics
    (C) Outpatient management with 10-day course of an oral antibiotic such as cephalexin
    (D) Observation at home pending results of blood cultures

Questions 446–448

Kara is a 13-month-old female who presents today for a well-child examination. Kara began walking approximately 6 weeks prior to this appointment. Her parents have concerns "about how bowlegged she is." Physical examination reveals a healthy toddler with symmetrical bowing below the knees. There are no obvious deformities and there is full ROM of the lower extremities.

446. Differential diagnosis in a child with bowleg deformity includes

    (A) Physiologic bowing
    (B) Blount disease
    (C) Rickets
    (D) All of the above

447. Which of the following information would be most helpful in determining the cause of this child's bowleg deformity?

    (A) Nutrition history
    (B) Family history of bowing
    (C) History of limb trauma or infection
    (D) All of the above

448. Appropriate management of this toddler would include

    (A) X-rays of lower extremities
    (B) Referral to an orthopedist
    (C) Measurement of the degree of bow-leggedness and reevaluation at her 18-month well-child examination
    (D) Bracing of the lower extremities

Questions 449–451

Kent is a 3-year-old male whose parent reports that he will not use his left arm today. Earlier in the day, the parent witnessed Kent's 7-year-old brother swinging Kent by his arms. It was shortly thereafter that the parent noted that Kent would not use his left arm. The brother denies a fall or direct trauma to the arm. In the office, Kent holds his forearm in a pronated position and will not use the arm. He actively resists attempts to flex it. His right arm has fully intact neurovascular status, is nontender, and has no apparent deformity or swelling.

449. Differential diagnosis of injuries involving the elbow region in preschool-age children includes

(A) Supracondylar fracture of the distal humerus
(B) Subluxation of the radial head
(C) Clavicle fracture
(D) All of the above

450. Based on this child's history and examination, the most likely diagnosis for this toddler is

(A) Subluxation of the radial head
(B) Acute tendinitis
(C) Fracture of the radial head
(D) Supracondylar fracture of the distal humerus

451. Treatment consists of

(A) X-ray of the left elbow and contralateral joint
(B) Hypersupination of the forearm with the elbow held in flexion
(C) X-ray of the left elbow, posterior splinting of left arm, and immediate referral to orthopedic surgery
(D) Observation at home only with follow-up in 24 hours

Questions 452–456

Kevin is a 14-year-old male who presents today with knee pain. The pain has evolved slowly and is local-

ized to the area below his right knee. There has been no direct trauma to the area and no recent fevers or illnesses. He plays interleague basketball year round. He has no pain at rest but it is exacerbated by running. There is no history of fever and he is afebrile at this visit. Physical examination reveals a normal ligament examination bilaterally. He has pain, tenderness, and swelling localized to the tibial tubercle below the knee bilaterally, right > left.

452. Differential diagnosis for this adolescent's proximal tibia pain would include

(A) Osteosarcoma
(B) Osteochondritis dissecans
(C) Baker's cyst
(D) Sever's disease

453. The most likely cause of this adolescent's knee pain would be

(A) Osteosarcoma
(B) Osgood-Schlatter disease
(C) Stress fracture of the proximal tibia
(D) Grade 1 or mild ligamentous injury of the knee

454. All the following are components of home management of simple musculoskeletal injuries and ligamentous sprains EXCEPT

(A) Rest
(B) Ice
(C) Casting
(D) Elevation

455. Which of the following statements regarding Osgood-Schlatter disease is *true*?

(A) Treatment always requires long-leg casting.
(B) Pain worsens with activity.
(C) Prominence of the tibial tuberosity will not persist into adulthood.
(D) It occurs most frequently in males and females 6–10 years old.

456. The most appropriate management of this adolescent's knee pain would be

(A) Nonweight bearing and referral to orthopedist for casting
(B) No specific treatment as pain will resolve at end of growth spurt
(C) Decrease or restriction of the activity that is exacerbating pain
(D) Restriction of activity for 48 hours, then may resume normal schedule

Questions 457–459

Shelly is a 12-year-old female who is seeing you today for her yearly well-child examination. Shelly's parent reports that the school nurse sent home a notice recently that Shelly was evaluated for scoliosis and that they "found a little curve." There has been no past medical or family history of scoliosis or orthopedic problems.

457. Scoliosis is defined as

(A) Anterior convex curvature of the spine
(B) Posterior convex curvature of the spine
(C) Lateral curvature of the spine
(D) None of the above

458. The most common type of scoliosis in all age groups is

(A) Functional scoliosis
(B) Idiopathic scoliosis
(C) Congenital scoliosis
(D) Neuromuscular scoliosis

459. Clinical presentation of idiopathic scoliosis typically includes all of the following EXCEPT

(A) Asymmetry of shoulder heights
(B) Back pain
(C) Waistline asymmetry
(D) Scapular prominence

ANSWERS AND RATIONALES

429. **(D)** Limp in children is never a normal symptom and requires further evaluation as to its cause. Trauma is the leading cause of painful limp in children of all ages. Slipped capital femoral epiphysis (SCFE) occurs as a result of repetitive microtrauma to the proximal femoral growth plate and is seen most commonly in very tall or very obese adolescents. Benign malignant neoplasms may cause a painful limp either due to the lesion itself or secondary to injury to surrounding bone (Renshaw, 1995). Duchenne's muscular dystrophy is a genetic disorder that results in progressive weakness and atrophy of specific muscle groups and causes a painless limp.

430. **(A)** In evaluating a child with a limp, laboratory tests are dictated by the history and physical findings. A complete blood count and erythrocyte sedimentation rate are useful screening tests in cases where systemic disease and/or infection may be suspected (Brady, 1993). Hip radiographs may be useful in determining the cause of the pain or limp (Tolo & Wood, 1993). In cases where it is difficult to distinguish septic arthritis from severe transient synovitis, aspiration of the hip joint may be necessary (Renshaw, 1995).

431. **(B)** Based on this child's health history, physical examination, diagnostic tests, and non-toxic appearance, the most likely diagnosis is transient synovitis. Transient synovitis is an acute inflammation of the hip, occuring most often in males and most commonly at ages 2–10 years. Transient synovitis often follows a viral URI or trauma, but the exact cause is unknown. All symptoms have a rapid onset and children are usually not systemically ill. Laboratory and hip x-rays are normal. The greatest concern is to rule out septic arthritis, a bacterial joint infection. Legg-Calvé-Perthes disease is an avascular necrosis of the femoral head common in males age 4–8 years, which occasionally can follow a course of toxic synovitis (Renshaw, 1995).

432. **(C)** The symptoms of transient synovitis are self-limiting and usually resolve within 3–5 days. Home management consists of rest, analgesics, and restricting activity in addition to daily telephone follow-up with the primary care provider during the course of illness.

433. **(A)** Metatarsus adductus is a congenital anomaly in which the forefoot is adducted with respect to the hindfoot and can be supple or fixed. In metatarsus adductus, the forefoot can be actively corrected with digital stimulation to the lateral border of the foot. Pes planus is also known as flatfoot and is not a cause of in-toeing. Femoral anteversion is a torsional deformity that occurs at the level of the hip, causing an in-toeing gait. Talipes equinovarus (clubfoot) is a congenital in-toeing anomaly of the foot consisting of three associated deformities—plantar flexion of the ankle, inversion of the heel, and forefoot adduction—that can be associated with neuromuscular abnormalities, such as spina bifida.

434. **(C)** Supple metatarsus adductus resolves spontaneously with growth in 90% of children (Craig & Goldberg, 1993). The etiology is assumed to be secondary to position of the intrauterine fetal foot. Internal tibial torsion is frequently present along with metatarsus adductus. In cases of supple metatarsus adductus, corrective shoes are generally not needed.

435. **(D)** For supple metatasus adductus, forefoot stretching exercises tid are taught to caregivers and may help to expedite resolution of the adduction. If the deformity fails to correct with stretching or spontaneously by 4 months of age, referral to an orthopedist for further evaluation is necessary (Craig & Goldberg, 1993).

436. **(D)** Internal tibial torsion is rotation of the leg between the knee and ankle, causing in-toeing. It is most commonly diagnosed between the ages of 6 months and 2 years and is thought to be secondary to molding due to intrauterine position (Tolo & Wood, 1993). It is present at birth and is not a progressive deformity. Femoral anteversion is the most common cause of in-toeing after age 3 years. It produces excessive internal rotation of the femur as compared with external rotation and and there is failure to progress to the normally anteverted position. Genu varum (bowleg) is normal from infancy through 2 years and is not a cause of in-toeing. Genu valgum (knock-knee) is considered a normal finding after age 2 years up to 8 years of age and is not a cause of in-toeing.

437. **(D)** Based on history, physical examination, and evaluation of the thigh–foot angle, the most likely cause of this toddler's in-toeing is internal tibial torsion.

438. **(C)** Growth alone corrects the vast majority (99%) of cases of internal tibial torsion by age 3–4 years (Sponseller, 1997). Improvement in the internal torsion is slowed in children who sleep prone because the feet are internally rotated during sleep (Tolo & Wood, 1993). Corrective shoes and night splints currently are thought to be of no real value or benefit.

439. **(B)** Although only 2–3% of all newborns present breech, 16–25% of DDH patients are born breech. Associated factors include family history of DDH, first-born infants, talipes equino-

varus, and metatarsus adductus (Novacheck, 1996). The incidence of DDH varies with race, with an increased incidence in Native American populations and a decreased incidence in African-American and Asian populations.

440. **(A)** Diagnosis of DDH in the newborn is made primarily by physical examination. Both the Barlow and Ortolani manuevers should be used to examine each hip individually (Figures A440a and b, p. 149). All newborns should have a hip examination and, if normal, it should be repeated at each well-baby visit through age 12 months (Aronsson, Goldberg, Kling, & Roy, 1994). DDH is four times more likely in females than in males and its etiology is multifactorial (genetic, mechanical, and/or physiologic) (Novacheck, 1996).

441. **(D)** The goal of early detection and treatment of DDH is to restore the articulation of the femur within the acetabulum, allow for normal bony development, prevent avascular necrosis, and shorten the course of treatment (Aronsson et al., 1994; Rudy, 1996).

442. **(C)** For newborns 0–6 months of age, the mainstay choice of treatment is generally the Pavlik harness (Aronsson et al., 1994; Novacheck, 1996). Triple-diapering is not advised as it promotes hip extension. For infants older than 6 months of age or who have not responded to Pavlik therapy, preliminary traction followed by closed reduction and spica casting are generally recommended (Aronsson et al., 1994). In severe cases, or in older children, open surgical reduction may be required to relocate the hip.

443. **(C)** Osteomyelitis is an infection of bone, most commonly of bacterial origin. Trauma is often a precipitating factor. The femur and tibia are the most common sites of infection in children, although any bone can be affected. Osteomyelitis must be differentiated from trauma, inflammatory joint diseases such as juvenile rheumatoid arthritis (JRA), cellulitis, joint infections, and age-related muscoloskeletal problems such as slipped capital femoral epiphysis (SCFE) and Legg-Calvé-Perthes disease. Muscoloskeletal tumors including Ewing's sarcoma and osteogenic sarcoma as well as leukemia may present with similar symptoms, limp, and limb swelling. In particular, Ewing's sarcoma may present as osteomyelitis or septic joint with fever and elevated WBC/ESR counts (Jackman, 1994).

444. **(B)** The most common bacterial pathogen is *Staphlococcal aureus* in all age groups, followed by gram-negative rods, group A streptococcus, and *H. influenzae* (rare now owing to effective vaccines). *Pseudomonas aeruginosa* remains an important cause of osteomyelitis in the foot, especially if a puncture wound occurred through a sneaker, where the bacteria are harbored in the spongy sole material. Salmonella is an important pathogen in children with hemoglobinopathies (Sponseller, 1997).

445. **(B)** Immediate orthopedic referral for evaluation, hospitalization, and IV antibiotics is warranted. In addition, radionucleotide imaging studies may be helpful in the early stage of diagnosis. Mortality from osteomyelitis is rare; however, delay in diagnosis or inadequate treatment can result in infection involving the epiphysis, increasing the risk for leg-length discrepancies.

446. **(D)** Physiologic bowleg (genu varum) in the newborn and infant is due to intrauterine positioning of the lower extremities. When the infant begins to stand and walk, this physiologic state begins to correct itself, usually by 18–24 months of age. Blount disease (tibia vara) is considered a pathologic genu varum. It is considered in the differential diagnosis of those infants and children whose genu varum does not begin to decrease in the second year of life, is asymmetrical, or is rapidly progressing. Rickets occurs when there is deficient mineralization of the maturing skeleton. The most common cause worldwide is a deficiency in dietary vitamin D. In the United States, the most common cause is familial hypophosphatemia.

447. **(D)** In assessing the child with genu varum, obtain a health history that includes assessment of the infant's or child's nutrition history, family history of bowlegs, history of limb trauma or infection, age of onset of bow-leggedness, and at what age the child began to stand and to walk.

448. **(C)** As the most likely cause of this toddler's genu varum is physiologic, the most appropriate management at this time is measurement of the degree of bowleggedness and re-evaluation by the primary care clinician at the 18-month well-child examination.

449. **(D)** Supracondylar fracture of the distal humerus is the most common fracture of the elbow. A fall on an outstretched hand with the elbow in extension is the common cause of this fracture. On a lateral x-ray of the elbow, a positive "fat pad" sign strongly suggests that a supracondylar fracture is present. Subluxation of the radial head is generally found in children under the age of 6 years and results from longitudinal traction to the wrist or forearm. Clavicle fracture is the most common fracture in young children. Commonly the child will not move the arm on the affected side secondary to pain.

450. **(A)** The most likely diagnosis based on the health history and physical examination is subluxation of the radial head, also known as "nursemaid's elbow." It generally occurs in children younger than age 6 years and results when the child's forearm or wrist is pulled with longitudinal force. Radiographs are normal.

451. **(B)** Subluxation of the radial head is generally reduced simply by supinating the forearm with the elbow held in flexion. Occasionally a small click may be felt when the radial head slips back under the annular ligament. Full movement of the arm and cessation of pain usually occurs immediately after reduction.

452. **(B)** Osteochondritis dissecans is a separation of a small portion of the femoral condyle with the overlying cartilage, often caused by a combination of trauma and ischemia of the bone. The patient is usually an adolescent with a 1–4-week history of nonspecific knee pain and swelling. A Baker's cyst presents with localized popliteal pain secondary to a herniation

of the synovium of the knee. Sever's disease is a common cause of heel pain in active children secondary to repetitive microtrauma at the insertion site of the achilles tendon on the calcaneus. Osteosarcoma is the most common pediatric primary malignancy of bone. It occurs most commonly in the distal femur of a teenager and shows a slight male tendency. The typical clinical picture is a teenager with a 3-month history of knee pain that is worse at night, unrelated to activity, with history of trauma to the knee area often only an incidental finding (Jackman, 1994; Renshaw, 1995).

453. **(B)** Osgood-Schlatter disease is the result of repetitive microtrauma to the immature tibial tubercle. The tibial tubercle is the primary site of insertion of the knee extensor mechanism on the proximal tibia. It is related to the adolescent growth spurt and level of athletic activity, and occurs commonly in males 13–14 years of age and females 10–11 years of age. Physical examination reveals tenderness to palpation and soft tissue swelling over the tubercle.

454. **(C)** Most simple, uncomplicated musculoskeletal injuries and ligamentous sprains may be managed following the principles of RICE (**R**est, **I**ce, **C**ompression, **E**levation).

455. **(B)** The microfractures of Osgood-Schlatter disease occur as a result of repeated extension of the knee associated with increased activity. Inflammation at the site of injury follows, resulting in pain and tenderness.

456. **(C)** Treatment for Osgood-Schlatter disease consists of restriction of the activity that is exacerbating the pain as needed and an explanation of the self-limited nature of this condition.

457. **(C)** Scoliosis is defined as a lateral curvature of the spine, when the child is viewed in the frontal plane from either the back or front (Tolo & Wood, 1993).

458. **(B)** Most cases of scoliosis are idiopathic, but there are also congenital and neuromuscular causes. The cause of idiopathic scoliosis is unknown and accounts for about 80% of all cases of scoliosis (Tolo & Wood, 1993).

459. **(B)** Noting asymmetry of the trunk is the key to detection of scoliosis. Symmetry of shoulder height, scapular position, and symmetry of the waistline are assessed. The child should be assessed while standing erect and then examined in the forward-bending position. The examination in all ages should include evaluation of the chest wall, back, and lower extremities (Figure A459, p. 150).

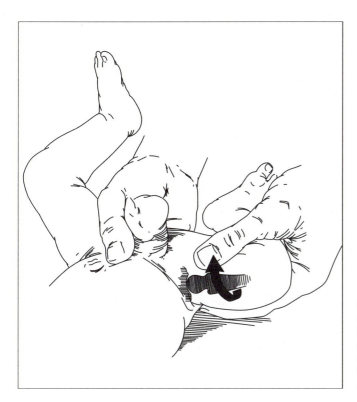

Figure A440a. Ortolani's test involves reduction of the dislocated hip by abduction in the flexed position. Examine only one hip at a time. This test is useful in children up to 3–5 months of age. *(Used with permission from Sponseller, P. D. (1997). Orthopedics. In B. J. Rosenstein & P.D. Fosarelli, eds.* Pediatric pearls: The handbook of practical pediatrics *(3d ed., p 264). St. Louis: Mosby.)*

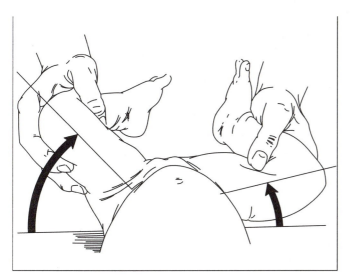

Figure A440b. In the older child with fixed dysplasia and in whom Barlow's and Ortolani's signs cannot be elicited, the main signs are limited abduction and apparent shortening. *(Used with permission from Sponseller, P. D. (1997). Orthopedics. In B. J. Rosenstein & P. D. Fosarelli, eds.* Pediatric pearls: The handbook of practical pediatrics *(3d ed., p. 265). St. Louis: Mosby.)*

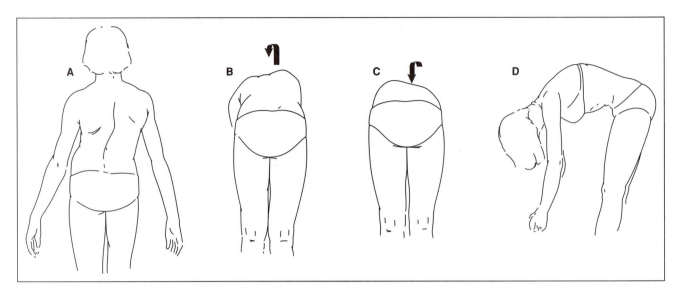

Figure A459. Screening for spinal deformities. **A.** Scoliosis may be demonstrated by subtle or striking elevation of one shoulder, a trunk shift, and waistline asymmetry. **B.** Forward bending with the hands clasped and the knees straight may reveal a thoracic prominence on the convex side, even if the standing exam appears normal. **C.** Further forward bending shows any lumbar curve (usually opposite of the thoracic curve). **D.** Always look from the side to see a focal kyphosis. *(Used with permission from Sponseller, P. D. (1997). Orthopedics. In B. J. Rosenstein & P. D. Fosarelli, eds. Pediatric pearls: The handbook of practical pediatrics (3d ed., p. 283) St. Louis: Mosby.)*

Infectious Diseases

Questions 460–463

Carlos is a 12-month-old child who is new to your practice. He presents today with his adoptive parents for his first well-child examination since arriving in the United States from his native country of Peru.

460. The current recommendations for skin testing for tuberculosis in children are based

   (A) On the age of the child
   (B) On assessment of the child's risk of exposure to tuberculosis
   (C) On the child's gender
   (D) All of the above

461. Which of the following skin tests is the "gold standard" for diagnosing tuberculosis infection in asymptomatic individuals?

   (A) Mantoux
   (B) Tine
   (C) Mono-Vacc
   (D) Aplitest

462. The most common clinical findings in children with tuberculosis include which of the following?

   (A) Sudden onset of high fever and cough
   (B) Frequent productive cough and low-grade fever
   (C) The majority of children are asymptomatic
   (D) Persistent fatigue

463. Commonly used chemotherapeutics for the treatment of TB in children include all the following EXCEPT

   (A) Isoniazid
   (B) Rifampin
   (C) Pyrazinamide
   (D) Ceftriaxone

Questions 464–468

Peter is a 9-year-old child who presents to your office today with a rash on his arm. The rash began on his right arm with a red papule approximately 3 weeks ago and over the past several days has grown to form a large annular lesion. There has been no history of trauma or bites to the area. Immunizations are up to date. He denies fever, fatigue, vomiting, or headache. His family recently vacationed along the Maryland coast. Physical examination is entirely normal except for this rash.

464. The most likely diagnosis for this patient is

   (A) Tinea corporis
   (B) Lyme disease
   (C) Pityriasis rosea
   (D) Erythema multiforme

465. The most likely causative agent in this 9-year-old's illness is

   (A) *Trichophyton rubrum*
   (B) *Treponema pallidum*
   (C) *Borrelia burgdorferi*
   (D) *Candida albicans*

466. All of the following may be early clinical manifestations of Lyme disease EXCEPT

(A) Fatigue
(B) Erythema migrans
(C) Splenomegaly
(D) Chronic arthritis

467. The antibiotic treatment most appropriate for this child with no known allergies would be

(A) Topical antifungal cream
(B) Doxycycline
(C) Penicillin VK
(D) Erythromycin

468. The best preventive measure against Lyme disease is

(A) Chemoprophylaxis in all children after a recognized deer tick bite
(B) Vaccination against Lyme disease
(C) Avoidance of tick-infested areas whenever possible
(D) All of the above

Questions 469–473

Suzanne is a 21-month-old toddler who has had a fever spiking to 39.4°C (103°F) for the past 5 days. She was seen at the clinic 3 days earlier when her temperature was 38.3°C (101°F). She was started on trimethoprim-sulfamethoxazole for a left acute otitis media. Today Suzanne is febrile 39.4°C (103°F) and appears ill. She has been irritable at home with decreased appetite and activity. On physical examination, she has a scarlatiniform rash in her groin area, red fissured lips, bright red tongue, and swollen cervical nodes.

469. Differential diagnosis for this toddler would include

(A) Scarlet fever
(B) Drug reaction/Stevens-Johnson syndrome

(C) Measles
(D) All of the above

In addition to the above findings, you note that the child has bilateral injected conjunctivas without history of discharge. Her immunizations are UTD and she has no known allergies.

470. The most likely diagnosis for this child is

(A) Stevens-Johnson syndrome
(B) Kawasaki syndrome
(C) Scarlet fever
(D) Rocky Mountain spotted fever

471. The most likely causative agent in Kawasaki syndrome is

(A) Rickettsial
(B) Viral
(C) A nontypical bacteria
(D) Unknown

472. Treatment of Kawasaki syndrome consists of

1. Treatment with oral amoxicillin for 14–21 days
2. High-dose aspirin therapy
3. Intravenous immune globulin (IVIG)

(A) 1 only
(B) 2 only
(C) 1, 2, and 3
(D) 2 and 3

473. The most common and serious sequela of Kawasaki syndrome is

(A) Juvenile rheumatoid arthritis
(B) Inflammation of the coronary arteries
(C) Aseptic meningitis
(D) Sterile pyuria

ANSWERS AND RATIONALES

460. **(B)** The American Academy of Pediatrics recommends focusing tuberculin skin testing on children who are at increased risk of acquiring tuberculous infection and disease. Therefore, children without risk factors who reside in low-prevalence regions, including those children who are 1 year of age, do not need to have routine tuberculin skin testing (American Academy of Pediatrics, 1997).

461. **(A)** The major diagnostic tool used in determining the presence of tuberculous infection in the asymptomatic patient is the Mantoux tuberculin skin test administered intradermally. Multiple puncture tests such as the Mono-Vacc and Tine are popular due to their ease of administration. However, the exact dose of tuberculin introduced cannot be quantitated accurately; therefore, it is difficult to interpret and standardize the reaction size.

462. **(C)** The majority of children with tuberculosis are discovered through contact investigations of adults who have infectious tuberculosis. In most of these cases, the children have asymptomatic disease that would have escaped detection if the infected adult had not been identified.

463. **(D)** Isonazid, rifampin, and pyrazinamide are bactericidal antituberculous drugs that inhibit the multiplication of *M. tuberculosis,* halting progression of tuberculosis and preventing the complication of early disease.

464. **(B)** Lyme disease is the most common vector-borne disease in the United States and is transmitted by ixodid ticks. More than 90% of all cases occur in three regions: states along the Eastern Seaboard (between Virginia and Massachusetts), the area around the Great Lakes, and states in the Pacific Northwest (Moskowitz & Meissner, 1997).

465. **(C)** The ixodid tick becomes infected in its larval stage by the spirochete *Borrelia burgdorferi* when it feeds on small mammals such as the white-footed mouse. The disease is transmitted to humans during the tick's nymphal stage. Most cases of acute disease occur between May and September. Transmission of the spirochete depends on how long the tick is attached to the host. Attachment for 24–48 hours is less likely to result in transmission of the spirochete than if the tick is attached for 72 hours or more (Moskowitz & Meissner, 1997).

466. **(D)** As with other spirochetal infections, the clinical signs of Lyme disease occur in several stages that may or may not overlap or occur in all infected individuals. The early, localized stage is characterized by low-grade fever, erythema migrans, splenomegaly, headache, fatigue, regional lymphadenopathy, and arthralgias. Later stage disease may be manifested by chronic arthritis, cardiac disease (AV block), and cranial neuropathies.

467. **(B)** Treatment of Lyme disease is based on the clinical signs and stage of the disease. In early localized disease, children over age 8 years may be treated with doxycycline 100 mg orally bid for 14–21 days. Children younger than age 8 years may be treated with amoxicillin

25–50 mg/kg/day tid (maximum 2 g/day) for 14–21 days (AAP, 1997).

468. **(C)** The best preventive measure against Lyme disease is avoidance of tick-invested areas. In tick-infested areas, clothing should cover as much of the arms and legs as possible. Daily inspection of the skin and prompt removal of ticks is also recommended. Prophylactic antibiotic treatment following a tick bite is not routinely indicated even in highly endemic areas (AAP, 1997).

469. **(D)** The signs and symptoms exhibited by this 21-month-old toddler may be clinically manifested in illnesses such as scarlet fever, Stevens-Johnson syndrome, and measles.

470. **(B)** Kawasaki syndrome is a febrile, multisystem, exanthematous illness. It occurs predominantly in children younger than age 5 years, occurs worldwide, and affects children of all races, with Asians at highest risk and Caucasians apparently at lowest risk (Rowley & Shulman, 1995).

471. **(D)** The clinical findings and epidemiology of Kawasaki syndrome "suggests that this syndrome may be caused by an infectious agent that leads to an immune-mediated syndrome in certain genetically predisposed individuals" (Rowley & Shulman, 1995). However, the cause of Kawasaki syndrome remains unknown.

472. **(D)** Management of Kawasaki syndrome is targeted at detecting coronary artery disease and early initiation of supportive care and anti-inflammatory therapy. Current recommended therapy for acute-stage Kawasaki syndrome includes intravenous immune globulin and high-dose aspirin therapy.

473. **(B)** The most common and serious sequela of Kawasaki syndrome is inflammation of the coronary arteries. Echocardiographic and angiocardiographic data have shown that approximately 20–25% of untreated children with Kawasaki syndrome develop coronary artery abnormalities, including aneurysms (Rowley & Shulman, 1995).

Genetic Issues

CASES AND QUESTIONS

Questions 474–478

Raylene is a 12-day-old infant girl born to a 32-year-old G2, P1 mother. She was born at 38.5 weeks, weighing 5 lb 7 oz. There were no complications during labor and delivery. On exam in the nursery, the infant was found to have the features typical of Turner's syndrome and therefore was referred to the geneticist for cytogenetics studies. Raylene's mother has come to the clinic for a well-child check.

474. In counseling the mother during the visit, you tell her Raylene is at risk for which of the following disorders?

    (A) Volvulus
    (B) Coarctation of the aorta
    (C) Wilms' tumor
    (D) Seizures

475. Physical manifestations of Turner's syndrome in children include

    (A) Webbed neck, short stature, cubitus valgus
    (B) Hypertelorism, low-set ears, situs inversus
    (C) Microagnathia, hip dysplasia, umbilical hernia
    (D) Microcephaly, cubitus valgus, pigmented nevi

476. Raylene should be monitored during health supervision visits for which of the following medical complications?

    (A) Serous otitis
    (B) Idiopathic hypertension
    (C) Obesity
    (D) All of the above

477. Which of the following statements is *true* concerning growth in children with Turner's syndrome?

    (A) They have similar growth patterns to unaffected children.
    (B) They have delayed growth patterns compared to unaffected children.
    (C) They have earlier growth acceleration than unaffected children.
    (D) They have accelerated growth patterns compared to unaffected children.

478. Children in middle childhood with Turner's syndrome may manifest which of the following?

    (A) Precocious puberty
    (B) Learning difficulties
    (C) Hyperthyroidism
    (D) None of the above

Questions 479–481

Jeff is brought in by his parents for routine care at 4.5 years of age. He has fragile X syndrome and is followed by the Genetics Disorder Clinic at the local teaching hospital.

479. The pattern of inheritance of fragile X syndrome is

(A) Autosomal recessive
(B) Autosomal dominant
(C) X-linked
(D) None of the above

480. Physical manifestations of fragile X include

(A) Developmental delay, micropenis, micrognathia
(B) Mental retardation, renal agenesis, polydactyly

(C) Macrocephaly, hypotonia, developmental delay
(D) Mental retardation, prominent forehead, macro-orchidism

481. Anticipatory guidance for this child with fragile X syndrome should include

(A) Behavioral intervention for hyperactivity
(B) Genetic counseling for family members at risk
(C) Review of the educational plan
(D) All of the above

ANSWERS AND RATIONALES

474. **(B)** Congenital malformations associated with Turner's syndrome include cardiac abnormalities such as coarctation of the aorta, bicuspid aortic valve, and aortic valve stenosis. An echocardiogram should be obtained and referral to a pediatric cardiologist should be made for any abnormalities on echocardiogram (American Academy of Pediatrics, 1995).

475. **(A)** Clinical findings associated with Turner's syndrome are short stature, webbed neck, low posterior hair line, cubitus valgus, and nail dysplasia. In addition to these physical manifestations, most females have delayed puberty and menarche as well as infertility (AAP, 1995; Castiglia, 1997).

476. **(D)** Children with Turner's syndrome require ongoing evaluation for some medical complications associated with this condition. Common abnormalities include cardiac disorders such as coarctation of the aorta, renal abnormalities such as horseshoe kidney, hearing loss related to serous otitis media, and obesity (AAP, 1995).

477. **(B)** Turner's syndrome is characterized by slight intrauterine growth retardation, a normal growth velocity for the first several years of life, and deceleration of growth later in childhood. These children also lack a pubertal growth spurt. Therapeutic trials of growth hormone have been used during childhood and puberty to increase height velocity and to help them achieve their anticipated adult height (Castiglia, 1997).

478. **(C)** Children with Turner's syndrome are not mentally retarded but may manifest learning disabilities that are described as a deficit in nonverbal or spatial ability. This difficulty can lead to frustration, poor self-esteem, and depression (Castiglia, 1997). Additionally, children with nonverbal learning disabilities may have behavioral problems in the social and emotional realms.

479. **(C)** Fragile X is a disorder in which the abnormal gene is carried by the long arm of the X chromosome. It is recognized as the most common hereditary cause of mental retardation, accounting for 30–50% of cases of X-linked mental retardation (Sujansky, Stewart, & Manchester, 1997).

480. **(D)** Distinctive physical features associated with fragile X syndrome in males include developmental delay or mental retardation, a prominent forehead, a prominent jaw, a dysmorphic face, and macro-orchidism. Other features include cleft palate, strabismus, serous otitis, orthopedic abnormalities, seizure disorders, and mitral valve prolapse (AAP, 1996).

481. **(D)** Health supervision of this child with fragile X syndrome should include discussing the need for behavioral interventions, reviewing the child's developmental and educational plan, and providing genetic counseling regarding the recurrence risk and prenatal diagnosis.

Miscellaneous Diseases and Disorders

CASES AND QUESTIONS

Questions 482–485

Kathy, a 15-month-old female, is here for a routine health supervision visit. The parental concern at this visit is the child's "small size." She was a term vaginal delivery, with both her weight and height at the 15th percentiles. The mother had an uneventful pregnancy, attended regular prenatal visits, and had no recorded history of alcohol, drug, or tobacco abuse. Kathy has been physically healthy and her developmental history has been normal to date. The father does not live with the family and he provides no monetary or emotional assistance. The mother is currently on public assistance. Today's physical examination and developmental screening are entirely normal. At the 12-month-exam, this child's weight was in the 10th percentile. Today's weight has fallen below the 5th percentile. Head circumference at all visits has been normal.

482. A clinical assessment in the child with potential failure to thrive (FTT) includes all of the following EXCEPT

(A) Assessment of developmental milestones and administration of the Denver Developmental Screening Test II
(B) Hospitalization of all children for observation and detailed assessment of feeding patterns
(C) Assessment of the child's nutritional status including review of growth parameters
(D) Complete health history, including family history, pre/postnatal history, and complete physical examination

483. Nonorganic failure to thrive

(A) Can be seen in children with cystic fibrosis
(B) Is characterized by deceleration of weight gain and delayed acquisition of developmental milestones
(C) Is the cause of failure to thrive in about 25% of all cases
(D) None of the above

484. Identified risk factors for nonorganic failure to thrive include all of the following EXCEPT

(A) Lead poisoning
(B) Parental neglect
(C) Underfeeding
(D) Inadequate caloric intake

After a thorough investigation of Kathy' nutritional, physical, and psychosocial history, it is determined that she has a mild-to-moderate failure to thrive without a discernible organic cause secondary to underfeeding and poor access to food.

485. Initial management of Kathy's FTT may include all of the following EXCEPT

(A) Immediate hospitalization
(B) Parenting education and nutritional recommendations/support
(C) Referral to social worker and support services such as WIC
(D) Close follow-up until normal growth is established

Questions 486–489

Joseph is a 15-month-old male who is here for a health supervision visit. The parent's chief complaint at this visit is his frequency of lower respiratory infection. His mother notes "that since birth, he always seems like he is sick." Joseph has had two episodes of pneumonia and two episodes of bronchiolitis, two of which required hospitalization. He has recently recovered from an uneventful course of varicella. At today's visit you note a steady decline in his weight-to-height ratio. He has a hearty appetite at home. He has loose, mucousy stools on the average of 2–3 times/day. He is a full-term healthy infant of a gravida 1, para 1 Caucasian mother. He has had sick visits on the average of 1/month for episodes of wheezing. Today he is well-appearing, slender, and in no apparent distress. He has a RR of 34/min with no retractions or flaring, a congested cough with rare scattered crackles, and wheezes bilaterally. His abdomen is nontender, soft, with active bowel sounds and no organomegaly. Additional PE is entirely normal. He attends family day care 2 days/week.

486. You have concerns about this child's history of frequent lower respiratory infections and decline in weight. Based on the history obtained, differential diagnoses for this child might include

(A) Cystic fibrosis
(B) Intestinal malabsorption
(C) Asthma
(D) All of the above

487. The clinical test accepted as the "gold standard" for the diagnosis of cystic fibrosis is

(A) Genetic testing for the CF gene using direct DNA analysis
(B) Quantitative pilocarpine iontophoretic sweat test
(C) Chest radiograph
(D) Spirometry

488. Cystic fibrosis is an autosomal recessive genetic disorder. For a child to have CF

(A) Only the female parent passes a CF gene on to the child.
(B) Both parents must pass a CF gene on to the child.
(C) Only the male parent passes a CF gene on to the child.
(D) None of the above.

Joseph has been diagnosed with cystic fibrosis (CF). The management of CF focuses on the maintenance of adequate growth and development and minimalization of symptoms, particularly progressive lung disease. He has been referred to a hospital with a CF treatment center. Joseph will continue to be followed by his primary care clinicians as primary care and well-child concerns continue to be an important part of his care.

489. In addition to a routine pediatric immunization schedule, it is recommended that children with CF receive which of the following immunizations?

(A) Pneumococcal vaccine
(B) Hepatitis A vaccine
(C) Varicella vaccine
(D) Meningococcal vaccine

Questions 490–493

Today Alan, age 8 years, presents to your office after falling down a hill while rollerblading. He was wearing a bicycle helmet and other protective gear and appears to have sustained only minor abrasions. Alan's mother states that since his last well-child visit 9 months ago, and also throughout the academic year, Alan has become increasingly impulsive and engages in "risky behaviors." She reminds you that he has also been "a high-energy kid" both at school and at home. He is in the third grade, is an average student, and is easily distracted. At home he becomes easily frustrated when playing with friends or siblings. His distractibility and impulsivity have been discussed briefly with his classroom teacher. His parents state that they believe his behavior has been, in part, due to a change in schools this year and that his high energy level is "just what boys are like." Except for a few scrapes and bruises, Alan's PE and neurologic assessment are entirely normal. During the physical examination and history-taking, Alan politely answers your questions, but is very distracted by the activity of his 3-year-old male sibling, who is also in the examination room.

490. The hallmarks of attention deficit hyperactivity disorder (ADHD) include:

1. Inattention
2. Hyperactivity
3. Inappropriate behavior
4. Impulsivity
5. Lying
    - (A) All of the above
    - (B) 1 and 4 only
    - (C) 1, 2, and 4
    - (D) 2, 3, and 5

491. All of the following are characteristics of ADHD EXCEPT

- (A) Onset of symptoms after age 7 years
- (B) Talking excessively
- (C) Trouble organizing school work
- (D) Easily distracted from tasks

492. Differential diagnosis for ADHD may include

- (A) Hearing and/or vision impairments
- (B) Seizure disorders
- (C) Autism
- (D) All of the above

493. The most commonly used medication in the United States for treatment of ADHD is

- (A) Macrolide antibiotics
- (B) Stimulants
- (C) Antidepressants
- (D) Antipsychotics

ANSWERS AND RATIONALES

482. **(B)** A comprehensive history and meticulous physical examination of the the child with suspected failure to thrive is necessary. The history would include family history; developmental history; prenatal/birth/neonatal histories; psychosocial history; medical history; nutritional assessment, including feeding patterns and review of growth parameters; and review of systems.

483. **(B)** Failure to thrive (FTT) typically describes infants and young children whose weight is persistently below the 5th percentile for age on standardized growth charts, in the absence of constitutional delay, or if the weight drops more than two major percentile groups (Frank, Silva, & Needlman, 1993; Bithoney, Dubowitz, & Egan, 1992). Nonorganic FTT is defined as growth deficiency without a diagnosable medical etiology. Whether nonorganic or organic, there are often multiple factors or problems that contribute to FTT.

484. **(A)** Nonorganic FTT often results from a combination of psychological, cultural, and/or financial issues and the cause is not physiologic. Organic FTT is the result of a specific physiologic condition.

485. **(A)** Initial management of this child's nonorganic FTT might include parenting education, nutritional therapy/recommendations/support, referral to a social worker and support services such as WIC, and close follow-up until normal growth is established. The initial management plan should be closely monitored and reevaluated at frequent intervals.

486. **(D)** Cystic fibrosis (CF) is the most commonly inherited lethal disease among the Caucasian population, with an incidence of 1:3000 live births (Meghdadpour, 1997). It affects the exocrine glands particularly of the gastrointestinal tract, respiratory system, and reproductive system. Excessive secretions then obstruct ducts and airways, leading to pancreatic insufficiency, respiratory infections, and intestinal malabsorption. (See Table A486.)

487. **(B)** The "sweat test" remains the "gold standard" for diagnosis of CF. Families with a child suspected of having CF, usually following a positive sweat test, can have genetic testing performed for the CF gene, although this test cannot yet identify 100% of those affected individuals (Meghdadpour, 1997). Prenatal testing is also available for high-risk families.

488. **(B)** Cystic fibrosis is an autosomal recessive genetic disorder. For a child to have CF, both parents must pass a CF gene on to their offspring.

489. **(A)** Children age 2 years or older with chronic pulmonary disease such as CF should receive the 23-valent pneumococcal vaccine as they are at increased risk of acquiring systemic pneumococcal infections or serious disease if they become infected.

490. **(C)** The three major characteristics of ADHD are inattention, impulsivity, and hyperactivity. *The Diagnostic and Statistical Manual of Mental*

Disorders (DSM-IV) (4/e) categorizes ADHD into three subtypes: (1) inattentive, (2) hyperactive-impulsive, and (3) combination of inattentive/hyperactive-impulsive (Borowsky, 1996; American Psychiatric Association, 1994).

491. **(A)** According to DSM-IV criteria, the symptoms of ADHD must appear before age 7 years and persist for at least 6 months before this disorder can be diagnosed.

492. **(D)** DSM-IV criteria must be met and differential diagnoses ruled out to confirm ADHD. Symptoms of ADHD can be seen in a number of other conditions, including hearing and/or vision impairments, seizure disorders, autism, genetic disorders such as fragile X syndrome, thyroid dysfunction, Tourette's syndrome, learning disabilities, iron-deficiency anemia, lead poisoning, and psychological disorders. Co-morbidity can be very common in children with ADHD, with up to 44% of these children carrying another psychiatric diagnosis (Borowsky, 1996).

493. **(B)** Stimulants are the most widely used medications for ADHD in the United States. Methylphenidate (Ritalin), dextroamphetamine (Dexedrine), and pemoline (Cylert) have been shown to increase attention span, lower impulsivity and hyperactivity, and increase gross and fine motor coordination (Borowsky, 1996; Burns & Shelton, 1996). Treatment for ADHD is multifaceted, and medications should be used in conjunction with behavioral, family, and cognitive-behavioral management (Burns & Shelton, 1996).

TABLE A486. PRESENTING SIGNS OF PATIENTS WITH CYSTIC FIBROSIS

1. Respiratory
Chronic cough, wheezing
Persistent atelectasis
"Recurrent pneumonia"
Staphylococcal pneumonia
Pseudomonas aeruginosa pneumonia, sinusitis, or bronchitis
Clubbing
Bronchiectasis
Nasal polyps
Hemoptysis

2. Gastrointestinal/nutritional
Meconium ileus or plug syndrome
Small bowel atresia
Meconium peritonitis
Direct hyperbilirubinemia
Unexplained hepatomegaly, cirrhosis
Failure to thrive
Steatorrhea
Chronic diarrhea
Rectal prolapse
Bowel obstruction
Hypoalbuminemia
Vitamin A, E, or K deficiency

3. Other
Family history of CF
Aspermia
Skin "tastes salty"
Metabolic alkalosis
Hypoelectrolytemia
Heat stroke, exhaustion
Elevated intracranial pressure (vitamin A deficit)
Intracranial hemorrhage (vitamin K deficit)

Reprinted with permission from Kirchner, K., & Abman, S.H. (1997). Respiratory tract. In G.B. Merenstein, D.W. Kaplan, & A.A. Rosenberg, eds. Handbook of pediatrics (18th ed., p. 500) Stamford, CT: Appleton & Lange.

Trauma and Emergencies

Questions 494–497

You receive a telephone call from a parent who frantically reports that her 11-year-old daughter just sustained multiple wasp stings. The parent states that the child has approximately 4 stings with mild soft tissue swelling at the sites and is crying secondary to pain. The child is not itchy, there are no hives, and she has an easy swallow without pharyngeal swelling. You determine that the child is in no apparent distress.

494. The most likely diagnosis for this child is

   (A) Localized reaction to the wasp stings
   (B) Anaphylactic reaction to the wasp stings
   (C) Mixed reaction—localized and systemic
   (D) Moderate systemic reaction to the wasp stings

495. You advise the parent to

   (A) Apply cold compresses to the affected sites
   (B) Review signs of moderate to severe allergic reactions—go to EW immediately if any signs of systemic reaction
   (C) Remove stinger if visible
   (D) All of the above

The parent calls 4 hours later to report that one of the sites on the child's arm has now developed "a large amount of localized swelling." She has full ROM of her arm and hand. The area is fairly itchy and nontender. There is no urticaria and no difficulty with breathing or swallowing.

496. Which of the following would you add to the child's current management plan?

   (A) Advise that the child be seen immediately by primary care provider.
   (B) Tell parent to administer diphenhydramine (Benedryl) (1 mg/kg orally) now and elevate arm.
   (C) Refer to allergist for skin testing.
   (D) All of the above.

This child's parent states that in the past this child has had hypersensitivity reactions to spider bites, but has never had an anaphylactic reaction.

497. A moderate to severe reaction from the bite of a brown recluse spider is characterized by

   (A) Local tissue damage including necrosis accompanied by systemic reactions such as fever, nausea, vomiting, urticaria, and arthralgias
   (B) Severe pain at the site of the bite
   (C) Pain, swelling, and pruritus at the site of the bite
   (D) Severe muscle spasms, pain, and rigid abdomen

Questions 498–503

Daniel is a 14-month-old male who presents to your office with burns to his right hand after grabbing his mother's curling iron off the bathroom counter. He has two small burns on the palm of his hand, measuring 2 and 3 cm, respectively. Each area blanches and is erythematous with a large blister covering each site. His skin is otherwise clear. He is sitting in his parent's lap and appears to have minimal discomfort.

498. Thermal burns are classified by the depth of the injury. Michael's burns can be described as:

(A) Superficial burn
(B) Superficial partial-thickness burn
(C) Deep partial-thickness burn
(D) Full-thickness burn

499. The most common cause of burns in children is secondary to

(A) Contact with high-voltage wires
(B) Contact with low-voltage current
(C) Contact with chemically strong household cleaners
(D) Scalding by immersion or spills

500. The extent of this child's burn would by determined by

1. The distribution and pattern of the burn
2. Affected area of the body
3. Percentage of body surface affected
4. Etiology of the burn
    (A) All of the above
    (B) 1 and 4
    (C) 2 and 3
    (D) 3 and 4

501. When reviewing this child's history, it is important that you review

(A) Number of siblings in his family
(B) Date of the last well-child examination
(C) Current immunization status
(D) All of the above

502. All of the following are *true* regarding child abuse EXCEPT

(A) The abuser often tells conflicting stories of the cause of the injury.
(B) The most frequent victims of child abuse are adolescents.
(C) The risk factors for child abuse may include substance abuse, spousal abuse, or poor child-care/parenting skills.
(D) Injuries in children who experience physical abuse are the result of direct trauma inflicted on the child.

503. Management of this child's burn would include

(A) Immediate hospitalization
(B) Administration of an oral antibiotic
(C) Daily dressing changes initially to assess for proper healing and infection
(D) All of the above

Questions 504–508

The frantic parent of a 2-year-old calls to report that she "gave her daughter too much Tylenol by mistake." This ingestion took place approximately 10 minutes ago. The child weighs 26 lb (11.8 kg). Normal dosage for weight of acetaminophen (Tylenol) for this child is 15 mg/kg/dose (177 mg) and the child ingested three 80-mg chewable tablets. The child's activity level is normal and there has been no pallor or vomiting.

504. The goal of telephone triage of suspected poisonings is

(A) To obtain sufficient information regarding the poisoning to determine its seriousness
(B) To initiate any immediate treatment that may be needed
(C) To assess any home treatment given
(D) All of the above

Accidental poisonings are common in the pediatric population and their prevention is an essential part of health supervision.

505. When offering advice regarding poisoning prevention at health supervision visits, you should

(A) Instruct parents to call the Poison Control Center first, prior to initiating treatment such as syrup of ipecac.
(B) Instruct parents to keep all medications and toxic substances high out of reach and in a locked cabinet.
(C) Review the connection between their child's developmental stage and potential sources of poisoning.
(D) All of the above.

506. All the following are *contraindications* for use of syrup of ipecac EXCEPT

(A) Acetaminophen ingestion
(B) Ingestion of hydrocarbons
(C) A child with diminished gag reflex
(D) An infant less than 6 months of age

507. A serious consequence of acetaminophen toxicity is

(A) Seizure
(B) Hepatotoxicity
(C) Arrhythmias
(D) Abdominal pain

508. Clinical manifestations of phase one iron toxicity include all the following EXCEPT

(A) Tinnitus
(B) Metabolic acidosis
(C) Hemorrhagic gastroenteritis
(D) Hyperglycemia

Questions 509–512

Kristin is a 6-year-old female who is brought to the local emergency room after falling off her bike 30 minutes ago. The parent who witnessed the accident saw the child skid on some road dirt when coming down her driveway. She fell off the bike directly onto her face, breaking the fall with her hands. She was wearing a bicycle helmet at the time of the accident. She did not lose consciousness and cried immediately. Here at the EW she is alert and cooperative. She has an abrasion down the bridge of her nose and had bleeding from her mouth, which is now controlled. Her entire PE is normal except for the facial injuries

and point tenderness of the distal radius of her right wrist.

509. Which of the following will best facilitate reimplantation of an avulsed permanent tooth?

(A) Apply direct pressure to the tooth socket.
(B) Soak the tooth in cold milk.
(C) Wrap the tooth in a dry, sterile dressing.
(D) All of the above.

510. Which of the following is the most common cause of nosebleed in children?

(A) Foreign body
(B) Picking of the nose
(C) Accidental trauma
(D) Upper respiratory infection

511. A unique feature of a child's skeleton that affects the type and severity of an orthopedic injury as well as treatment and healing is

(A) Epiphyseal growth plate
(B) Ligamentous laxity
(C) Cartilaginous long bones
(D) None of the above

512. Emergency management of a suspected fracture would include

(A) Evaluation of neurologic status
(B) Evaluation of vascular status
(C) Stabilization of the child, including airway maintenance
(D) All of the above

ANSWERS AND RATIONALES

494. **(A)** Reactions to insect bites or stings may be categorized as local (redness, pain, and soft tissue swelling at the site) or systemic (urticaria, hypotension, wheezing, laryngeal edema, shock). Reactions, whether local or systemic, generally occur within 2 hours of the sting or bite.

495. **(D)** Treatment for local reactions includes applying cold compresses, stinger removal, and review of signs of moderate to severe allergic reaction.

496. **(B)** In addition to standard treatment for local insect reactions, an additional appropriate treatment of this moderate local reaction to a wasp sting would include an antihistamine such as diphenhydramine (Benedryl).

497. **(A)** The bite of a brown recluse spider begins with redness and swelling at the site. In moderate to severe cases, there is local tissue damage including necrosis accompanied by systemic reactions such as fever, nausea, vomiting, urticaria, and arthralgias.

498. **(B)** Thermal burns are classified by depth of injury. Superficial (first degree) burns involve only the epidermis. Partial-thickness (second degree) burns involve the epidermis and part of the dermis. Full-thickness (third degree) burns involve the epidermis, dermis, and dermal appendages. This child's superficial partial-thickness burn is characterized by erythema, blistering, sensitivity to air, swelling, and pain.

499. **(D)** In 1994, the National Safety Council identified fires and burns as the third leading cause of accidental death in ages 1–24 years. Although burns can be caused by chemical, electrical, or thermal agents, the major cause of burns in children is scalding by immersion or spills.

500. **(A)** The extent of a burn injury is determined by the distribution and pattern of the burn, the affected area of the body, percentage of body surface affected, and etiology of the burn.

501. **(C)** Immunization history should be reviewed and tetanus prophylaxis administered to those susceptible children with a burn.

502. **(B)** There are over 2 million reported cases of child abuse annually in the United States. Child abuse may take many forms, including sexual, physical, and emotional abuse. The most frequent victims of child abuse are children less than 3 years of age (Berkowitz, 1996).

503. **(C)** Management of this child's burn would initially include pain management and daily dressing changes to assess for proper healing and signs of infection.

504. **(D)** Often cases of ingestion come to attention via telephone call. The goal of telephone triage, therefore, is to obtain sufficient information regarding the poisoning to determine its seriousness, to initiate any immediate treatment needed, and to assess any home treatment given.

505. **(D)** Emphasis should be put on prevention as the best management for poisonings (Table A505). Anticipatory guidance should be age and developmentally appropriate, and the PNP should review the connection with the caregiver between the child's developmental stage and potential sources of poisoning. The caregiver should be instructed to keep all medications and toxic substances high out of reach and in a locked cabinet, and to call the Poison Control Center first before initiating home treatment such as syrup of ipecac.

506. **(A)** Parents should be instructed to call the Poison Control Center first before administering syrup of ipecac to a child. Contraindications for use of syrup of ipecac include ingestions of acids, alkalis, and hydrocarbons; ingestion of seizure-inducing drugs; ingestion of sharp objects; children with diminished gag reflex; coma; and infants less than 6 months of age.

507. **(B)** Acetaminophen, a pediatric analgesic-antipyretic, has now become one of the most common over-the-counter medications ingested by young children. In addition, it is also one of the 10 most common drugs used by adolescents in intentional self-poisoning (Henretig & Shannon, 1996). One of the more serious consequences of acetaminophen toxicity is hepatotoxicity.

508. **(A)** Clinical manifestations of iron toxicity are divided into four phases. Phase one iron toxicity, which occurs within 1 hour of ingestion, manifests itself with hemorrhagic gastroenteritis (vomiting and bloody diarrhea), metabolic acidosis, and hyperglycemia.

509. **(B)** Avulsion is the term used to describe a tooth's total displacement from its socket. The appropriate management is to gently rinse the tooth under running water, being careful not to handle, scrub, or disturb the tooth's root. The ideal transport medium is milk; however, saline or saliva is also suitable and the tooth should be immediately reimplanted by a dentist within 30–60 minutes of the avulsion.

510. **(B)** Epitaxis is common in 4–10-year-olds and most commonly occurs in the anterior portion of the nasal septum. The most common cause of epitaxis is nose "picking." Other causes include trauma, inflammation, dryness, and crusting.

511. **(A)** Certain anatomic and physiologic differences in children's bones—such as the presence of the epiphyseal growth plate, greater skeletal plasticity, and a thicker periosteum—predispose them to different fracture patterns than those seen in adults. Fractures are classified based on anatomic location, type of fracture, and degree of displacement. The Salter-Harris classification is used most commonly to classify epiphyseal growth plate injuries. Approximately 15% of all fractures in children involve the growth plate.

512. **(D)** Emergency management of a suspected fracture in a child would include a complete history of the injury. Physical examination would include stabilization of the child, including airway management and evaluation of the neurologic status, musculoskeletal status, and vascular status of the affected extremity or part.

TABLE A505. SAFETY ISSUES AND PREVENTION STRATEGIES

Safety Issues	Prevention Strategies
Motor vehicle: (occupant, pedestrian bicycle)	Use child-restraint device that is age appropriate. Never leave child alone in car. Wear safety helmets appropriate for activity (bicycling, skateboarding, skating, horseback riding). Teach rules of pedestrian safety. Be a role model for appropriate behavior (eg, parents use seat belts, helmets).
Burns	Reduce hot water temperature. Purchase, install, and check smoke alarms and fire extinguishers. Use nonflammable clothing, toys, and household products. Avoid smoking.
Poisoning	Safely store drugs, cleaning agents, chemicals, and corrosives. Use child-resistant caps on drug containers. Keep syrup of ipecac in the home. Post poison control and emergency facility number by the phone.
Drowning	Supervise children around water. Lock gates around swimming pools. Teach water safety and swimming.
Play	Monitor safety of toys and activities.
Violence	Remove handguns from the home *or* lock all weapons and ammunition in separate areas. Assess family for substance abuse, child abuse, and family violence.
General	Provide education and guidance before child exhibits behaviors or skills that may lead to injury. Assess risk factors, environmental factors, and stress-related factors at each clinic visit.

Reprinted with permission from Eldridge, T.M. (1997). Injury prevention. In J.A. Fox, ed. Primary health care of children (p. 195). St. Louis: Mosby.

IV

Professional Issues

Professional Issues

CASES AND QUESTIONS

Questions 513–537

513. Which physician/nurse team was instrumental in developing the role of the nurse practitioner?

   (A) Henry Silver and Loretta Ford
   (B) John Smith and Mary Forest
   (C) Harold Sullivan and Rosemary Fromm
   (D) Ronald Sunog and Melissa Fillmore

514. According to the ANA Standards of Practice for the Primary Health Care Nurse Practitioner, which of the following statements is *true* regarding Scope of Practice?

   (A) It is divided into practice and performance categories.
   (B) It was developed in 1990 by the ANA to define the concepts of primary health care and the educational preparation and practice characteristics of the primary health care nurse practitioner.
   (C) It provides a means for evaluating, critiquing, and measuring the achievement of excellence for nurse practitioners in the primary health care setting.
   (D) It defines more clearly the role of the nurse practitioner as a primary health care provider.

515. Which nationwide legislative reform is *not* creating a barrier to practice by nurse practitioners?

   (A) Direct third-party reimbursement
   (B) Prescriptive writing authority
   (C) A Legal Scope of Practice
   (D) Autonomous practice

516. Which statement is *true* regarding comparison studies of physicians and nurse practitioners?

   (A) Physicians provide a much higher quality of health care in almost all categories.
   (B) Primary care provided by nurse practitioners is equivalent or superior to that provided by physicians.
   (C) There is virtually no difference in quality of health care when comparing physicians and nurse practitioners.
   (D) Nurse practitioners score higher in comprehensiveness, quality, and cost than physicians.

517. A patient's parent complains to you that your physician colleague is "very standoffish and doesn't pay attention to my child when he is examining him." Your *best* response would be to

   (A) Ignore what she said and continue your exam of the child.
   (B) Encourage her to talk to the physician and express her concerns in a nonthreatening manner.
   (C) Tell her you empathize with her but there really isn't anything you can do about it except listen.
   (D) Tell her you'll talk to the physician for her and explain her concerns.

518. The basic differences between health care provided by a nurse practitioner and that by a physician are

(A) A nurse practitioner evaluates the illness differently, placing the focus on why the patient is at a specific risk and emphasizing disease prevention, health promotion, and health maintenance.
(B) Physicians are more accurate with their diagnoses of medical problems and have more knowledge about medical treatments than nurse practitioners.
(C) Nurse practitioners have more task-oriented skills than a physician; therefore they provide more comprehensive care.
(D) Patients are more likely to listen to a physician than a nurse practitioner because physicians are perceived to have more medical knowledge.

519. Which statement *best* describes the level of authority and reimbursement for nurse practitioners?

(A) Level of authority and reimbursement varies from state to state.
(B) Forty states now authorize nurse practitioners to write prescriptions, although they differ widely in the degree of autonomy they grant.
(C) All states require strict supervision by physicians regarding both autonomy and perscriptive authority.
(D) Nurse practitioner authority is outlined specifically by the ANA, with reimbursement provided differently by each individual insurance company.

520. Which group has been identified as being the most reluctant to support the role of the nurse practitioner?

(A) AMA
(B) ANA
(C) Insurance companies
(D) HMOs

521. What type of practice has been identified as the best model, benefiting both physicians and nurse practitioners?

(A) Employment of nurse practitioners only by primary care physicians to minimize malpractice liability
(B) Utilizing the nurse practitioner for well-child and simple illnesses only and the physician for diagnosing and treating complex cases and managing critical and unstable medical conditions
(C) A nurse practitioner clinic using primary care physicians as consultants and referral sources
(D) A collaborative practice where nurse practitioners bear the principal responsibility for the diagnosis and management of uncomplicated illness and provide the education, counseling, and management of disease prevention and health promotion

522. Which statement is *true* in defining the requirements of advanced practice nurses?

(A) Advanced practice nurses can be any nurse licensed and certified, with long-term experience in a speciality area.
(B) Advanced practice nurses are registered nurses with specialty training, usually at a master's degree level, providing health care in both primary and acute care.
(C) Advanced practice nurses must have a master's degree and be licensed and certified in their area of expertise.
(D) Any person with a degree in any field can apply, train, and be certified as an advanced practice nurse.

523. Which study provided the most supportive evidence of the role of the nurse practitioner?

(A) Extensive meta-analysis by the ANA
(B) Research analysis compiled by the APA
(C) The 1986 Office of Technical Assessment (OTA) report
(D) The 1996 APN study by the American Academy of Nurse Practitioners

524. Which is the *best* statement regarding nurse practitioners and malpractice liability?

(A) Insurance premiums for nurse practitioners are increasing due to the expanding responsibility acquired in their role.

(B) Nurse practitioners are responsible for less than 1% of all malpractice claims.

(C) Insurance companies refuse third-party reimbursement to nurse practitioners because of the high liability of their role.

(D) Malpractice insurance premiums and the low incidence of malpractice claims indicate that patients are satisfied with nurse practitioner care.

525. Your supervising physician is hesitant about defining protocols for use in the office. The main reason protocols are so important is

(A) They provide guidelines for practice as defined and agreed upon by both the nurse practitioner and physician, based on current standards, practices, and research.

(B) They decrease the liability for the nurse practitioner.

(C) Protocols are not very helpful, especially if the supervising physician doesn't feel guidelines are necessary to define your practice.

(D) Protocols provide a framework for establishing practice guidelines and are not meant to be adhered to strictly.

526. The two most important findings by the Burlington Randomized Trial Study are

(A) That nurse practitioners rate high in consumer satisfaction and they provide a high quality of care

(B) That nurse practitioners provide primary care as safely and effectively as physicians and appropriate referrals were made when medical intervention was necessary

(C) That between 75 and 80% of adult primary care services and up to 90% of pediatric primary care services could be performed by nurse practitioners

(D) That patients respond more favorably to nurse practitioners and feel more comfortable asking questions thought to be too trivial to ask a physician

527. Which statement is most frequently used by physicians when expressing their concern regarding nurse practitioner–provided primary care?

(A) Nurse practitioners cannot perform tasks—ie, suturing, phlebotomy, IV placement—as well as physicians.

(B) Nurse practitioners use less invasive technology.

(C) Nurse practitioners have poor practice guidelines in providing primary care.

(D) Nurse practitioners have less experience in providing primary care because they have less training.

528. The following statements are true regarding the *support role* of the nurse practitioner EXCEPT

(A) The nurse practitioner participates as a team member in the provision of medical and health care, interacting with professional colleagues to provide comprehensive care.

(B) Nurse practitioners combine a number of roles to provide quality comprehensive health care.

(C) Some of the most important roles are those of provider, mentor, educator, and researcher.

(D) Nurse practitioners can also be utilized as managers and consultants.

529. Which tool is described as the Basis for Practice by the American Academy of Nurse Practitioners?

(A) Quality assurance

(B) Accurate documentation of client status and care

(C) The nursing process

(D) Research

530. The two most challenging health care problems facing the United States in this century and the future are

    (A) Rapidly rising medical costs and lack of medical coverage
    (B) Lack of medical insurance and lack of capable providers
    (C) A low rate of inflation and high medical costs
    (D) High unemployment and lack of qualified medical providers

531. According to the 1986 OTA Report, what potential benefits to health care do nurse practitioners provide?

    (A) An equivalent alternate choice to physicians and greater access to health care
    (B) Less likely to prescribe drug treatments and costly invasive diagnostic techniques
    (C) Increased access to care and decreased cost of health care
    (D) Potential societal benefits and an increase in cost

532. Which statement is *true* regarding direct reimbursement for nurse practitioners?

    (A) Nurse practitioners are mandated by Congress to receive all forms of direct reimbursement from all insurance providers.
    (B) Direct reimbursement of Medicaid and Medicare to nurse practitioners varies from state to state.
    (C) Currently nurse practitioners do not receive direct reimbursement of any kind.
    (D) Nurse practitioners do not need direct reimbursement because they bill under their supervising physician's provider number and receive 100% restitution.

533. What group defines the nurse practitioner's legal scope of practice?

    (A) ANA (American Nurses Association)
    (B) State Boards of Nursing
    (C) AANP (American Association of Nurse Practitioners)
    (D) Individual state nurses associations

534. The nurse practitioner provides, or provides for, health care that

    (A) Is comprehensive and continuous
    (B) Spans the health care continuum
    (C) Is coordinated with all aspects of primary care
    (D) All of the above

535. Nurse practitioner practice, based on research, results in

    (A) Improved health care outcomes
    (B) Further development of the role of the nurse practitioner
    (C) Delivery of optimum primary health care
    (D) An increase of knowledge and skill

536. What framework does the nurse practitioner use for managing patient care?

    (A) Research
    (B) Quality assurance
    (C) Policies and procedures
    (D) The nursing process

537. Studies have shown that nurse practitioners rate highest in

    (A) Proper diagnoses
    (B) Patient management
    (C) Patient care
    (D) Consumer satisfaction

ANSWERS

513. (A)

514. (D)

515. (C)

516. (B)

517. (B)

518. (A)

519. (A)

520. (A)

521. (D)

522. (B)

523. (C)

524. (D)

525. (A)

526. (B)

527. (D)

528. (A)

529. (D)

530. (A)

531. (C)

532. (B)

533. (B)

534. (D)

535. (A)

536. (D)

537. (D)

Bibliography

IMMUNIZATIONS

American Academy of Pediatrics. (1997). Active and passive immunization. In G. Peter (Ed.), *1997 Red book: Report of the Committee on Infectious Diseases (24th ed.,* pp. 1–68). Elk Grove, IL: American Academy of Pediatrics.

American Academy of Pediatrics. (1997). Hepatitis B. In G. Peter (Ed.), *1997 Red book: Report of the Committee on Infectious Diseases (24th ed.,* pp. 247–260). Elk Grove, IL: American Academy of Pediatrics.

American Academy of Pediatrics. (1997). Pneumococcal Infections. In G. Peter (Ed.), *1997 Red book: Report of the Committee on Infectious Diseases (24th ed.,* pp. 410–419). Elk Grove, IL: American Academy of Pediatrics.

American Academy of Pediatrics. (1997). Poliovirus Infections. In G. Peter (Ed.), *1997 Red book: Report of the Committee on Infectious Diseases (24th ed.,* pp. 424–433). Elk Grove, IL: American Academy of Pediatrics.

American Academy of Pediatrics. (1997). Varicella-zoster infections. In G. Peter (Ed.), *1997 Red book: Report of the Committee on Infectious Diseases (24th ed.,* pp. 573–585). Elk Grove, IL: American Academy of Pediatrics.

American Academy of Pediatrics. (1997). Appendix II: Standard for pediatric immunization practices. In G. Peter (Ed.), *1997 Red book: Report of the Committee on Infectious Diseases (24th ed.,* pp. 668–680). Elk Grove, IL: American Academy of Pediatrics.

Centers for Disease Control and Prevention. (1991). Hepatitis B virus: A comprehensive strategy for eliminating transmission in the United States through universal childhood vaccination. *MMWR, 40,* 1–17.

Colizza, D.F. (1995). Pertussis update. *Journal of School Health, 65(5),* 195–198.

Jenson, H.B., & Baltimore, R.S. (1995). *Pediatric infectious diseases: Principles and practices.* Stamford, CT: Appleton & Lange.

Moyer, M.S., & Jenson, H.B. (1995). Viral hepatitis. In H.B. Jenson & R.S. Baltimore, *Pediatric infectious diseases: Principles and practices* (pp. 1169–1188). Stamford, CT: Appleton & Lange.

Nowicki, M.J., & Balistreri, W.F. (1992). Hepatitis A to E: Building up the alphabet. *Contemporary Pediatrics, 9,* 118–128.

Nowicki, M.J., & Balistreri, W.F. (1992). The C's, D's, and E's of viral hepatitis. *Contemporary Pediatrics, 9,* 23–42.

Peterson, C.L., Vugia, D.J., Meyers, H.B., Chao, S.M., Vogt, J., Lanson, J., Brunell, P.A., Kim, K.S., & Mascola, L. (1996). Risk factors for invasive group A streptococcal infections in children with varicella: A case-control study. *Pediatric Infectious Disease Journal, 15(2),* 151–156.

Watson, B., & Haupt, R.M. (1997). Varicella vaccine: Removing the roadblocks. *Contemporary Pediatrics, 14(5),* 166–181.

GENERAL NUTRITION

American Academy of Pediatrics, Committee on Drugs. (1994). The transfer of drugs and other chemicals into human milk. *Pediatrics, 93,* 137–150.

American Academy of Pediatrics. (1993). *Pediatric nutrition handbook.* Elk Grove, IL: American Academy of Pediatrics.

American Academy of Pediatrics. (1995). Fluoride supplementation for children: Interim policy recommendations. *Pediatrics, 95(5),* 777.

Dennison, B.A., Rockwell, H.L., & Baker, S.L. (1997). Excess fruit juice consumption by preschool-aged children is associated with short stature and obesity. *Pediatrics, 99(1),* 15–22.

Felman, A.L. (1997). Breastfeeding. In C.E. Burns, N. Barber, M.A. Brady, & A.M. Dunn, *Pediatric primary care: A handbook for nurse practitioners* (pp. 259–276). Philadelphia: W.B. Saunders.

Gerber Products Company. (1995). Human milk and infant formula. *Current Practices in Infant Feeding,* 9–14.

Hether, N.W. (1998). Fluoride and dental public health. *Pediatric Basics, 82,* 1 & 11.

Mellin, L. (1992). *Report from the Center for Child and Adolescent Obesity: Child Obesity Recommendations for the United States* (pp 1–7). University of California, San Francisco.

Munoz, K.A., Krebs-Smith, S.M., Ballard-Barbash, R., & Cleveland, L.E. (1997). Food intakes of U.S. children and adolescents compared with recommendations. *Pediatrics, 100*(3), 323–329.

National Association of Pediatric Nurse Associates and Practitioners. (1993). NAPNAP position statement: Breast-feeding. *Journal of Pediatric Health Care, 7*(6), 289.

Trahms, C.M., & Pipes, P.L. (1997). *Nutrition in infancy and childhood* (6th ed.). Philadelphia: WCB/ McGraw-Hill.

Troiano, R.P., Flegal, K.M., Kuczmarski, R.J., Campbell, S.M., & Johnson, C.L. (1995). Overweight prevalence and trends for children and adolescents: The National Health and Nutrition Examination Surveys, 1963–1991. *Archives of Pediatric and Adolescent Medicine, 149,* 1085–1091.

Whitaker, R.C., Wright, J.A., Pepe, M.S., Seidel, K.D., & Dietz, W.H. (1997). Predicting obesity in young adulthood from childhood and parental obesity. *New England Journal of Medicine, 337*(13), 869–873.

GROWTH AND DEVELOPMENT

Abrams, R.B., & Mueller, W.A. (1997). Oral medicine and dentistry. In *Current pediatric diagnosis and treatment* (13th ed., Ch. 16, pp. 393–402). Stamford: Appleton & Lange.

American Academy of Pediatrics. (1995). Committee on Practice and Ambulatory Medicine: Recommendations for preventive pediatric health care. *Pediatrics, 96,* 373.

American Academy of Pediatrics. (1997). Sexually transmitted diseases. In G. Peter, ed. *1997 Red book: Report of the Committee of Infectious Diseases* (24th ed., pp. 108–112). Elk Grove Village, IL: American Academy of Pediatrics.

Andrews, John. (1997). Making the most of the sports physical. *Contemporary Pediatrics, 14*(3), 183–205.

Blum, Nathan, & Carey, William. (1996). Sleep problems among infants and young children. *Pediatrics in Review, 17*(3), 87–92.

Capute, Arnold, Shapiro, Bruce, & Palmer, Frederick. (1987). Marking the milestones of language development. *Contemporary Pediatrics, 4*(4), 24–41.

Cavanaugh, Robert. (1994). Anticipatory guidance for the adolescent: Has it come of age? *Pediatrics in Review, 15*(12), 485–489.

Chaikind, Janet, & Shafer, Mary-Ann. (1996). Breast problems. In *Rudolph's pediatrics* (20th ed., Ch 2.5.1, pp. 57–58). Stamford, CT: Appleton & Lange.

Charlton, Valerie, & Phibbs, Roderic. (1996). Examination of the newborn. In *Rudolph's pediatrics* (20th ed., Ch. 5.3, pp. 208–218). Stamford, CT: Appleton & Lange.

Coleman, William, & Howard, Barbara. (1995). Family-focused behavioral pediatrics. Clinical techniques for primary care. *Pediatrics in Review, 16*(12), 448–455.

Coupey, Susan, & Schonberg, S. Kenneth. (1997). Drug, alcohol and tobacco use. In Robert Hoekelman, ed. *Primary pediatric care* (3rd ed., Ch. 99, pp. 799–806). St. Louis: Mosby–Year Book.

Dixon, Suzanne. (1992). *Encounters with children: Pediatric behavior and development* (2nd ed.). St. Louis: Mosby–Year Book.

Dworkin, Paul. (1996). Screening. In Robert Hoekelman, ed. *Primary pediatric care* (3rd ed., Ch. 20, pp. 200–247). St. Louis: Mosby–Year Book.

Ehrman, Wendi. (1997). Obesity. In Robert Hoekelman, ed. *Primary pediatric care* (3rd ed., Ch. 234, pp. 1448–1452). St. Louis: Mosby–Year Book.

Frankenburg, William et al. (1992). The Denver Developmental Screening Tool II: A major revision and restandardization of the Denver Developmental Screening Tool. *Pediatrics, 89,* 91–97.

Goldenring, John, & Cohen, Eric.(1988). Getting into adolescent HEADSS. *Contemporary Pediatrics, 5,* 75–90.

Gundy, John. (1997). The pediatric physical exam. In Robert Hoekelman, ed. *Primary pediatric care* (3rd ed., Ch. 7. pp. 55–97). St. Louis: Mosby– Year Book.

Hagerman, Randi. (1997). Growth and development. In *Current pediatric diagnosis and treatment* (13th ed., Ch. 1, pp. 1–19). Stamford, CT: Appleton & Lange.

Headley, Roxann, & Lustig, James. (1997). Ambulatory pediatrics. In *Current pediatric diagnosis and treatment* (13th ed., Ch. 9, pp. 215–233). Stamford, CT: Appleton & Lange.

Howard, Barbara. (1990). Growing together. The toddler years need not be turbulent. *Contemporary Pediatrics, 7,* 21–40.

Irwin, Charles, Shafer, Mary-Ann, & Ryan, Sheryl. (1996). Health problems of adolescents. In *Rudolph's pediatrics* (20th ed., Ch. 2.2, pp. 40–44). Stamford, CT: Appleton & Lange.

Jenkins, Renee, & Saxena, Sunita. (1995). Keeping adolescents healthy. *Contemporary Pediatrics, 12*(6), 76–89.

Kulin, Howard, & Muller, Jorn. (1996). The biological aspects of puberty. *Pediatrics in Review, 17*(3), 75–86.

Mahoney, C. Patrick. (1990). Adolescent gynecomastia: Differential diagnosis and management. *Pediatric Clinics of North America, 37*(6), 1389–1401.

Maxson, Suzanne & Yamauchi, Terry. (1996). Otitis media. *Pediatrics in Review, 17*(6), 191–196.

Miller, Norman, & Cocores, James. (1993). Nicotine dependence: Diagnosis, chemistry and pharmacologic treatments. *Pediatrics in Review, 14*(7), 275–279.

Nowak, Arthur. (1993). What pediatricians can do to promote oral health. *Contemporary Pediatrics, 10*(4), 90–106.

Overby, Kim. (1996). Counseling and anticipatory guidance. In *Rudolph's pediatrics* (20th ed., Ch. 1.4, pp. 19–29). Stamford, CT: Appleton & Lange.

Pakula, Lawrence. (1992). Sibling rivalry. *Pediatrics in Review, 13*(2), 72–73.

Parkin, Patricia, Schwartz, Clive, & Manuel, Betty Ann. (1993). Randomized controlled trial of three interventions in the management of persistent crying of infancy. *Pediatrics, 92*(2), 197–201.

Perrin, Ellen. (1996). Pediatricians and gay and lesbian youth. *Pediatrics in Review, 17*(9), 311–318.

Prazar, Gregory. (1997). Lying and Stealing. In Robert Hoekelman, ed. *Primary pediatric care* (3rd ed., Ch. 84, pp. 734–736). St. Louis: Mosby–Year Book.

Schlossberger, Norman, Kogan, Barry, & Shafer, Mary-Ann. (1996). Scrotal masses. In *Rudolph's pediatrics* (20th ed., Ch. 2.5.2, pp. 58–60). Stamford, CT: Appleton & Lange.

Simm, M.D. (1991). Foster children and the foster care system II: Impact on the child. *Current Problems in Pediatrics, 21,* 345.

Smoyak, Shirley. (1997). Changing American Families. In Robert Hoekelman, ed. *Primary pediatric care* (3rd ed., Ch. 54, pp. 610–616). St. Louis: Mosby–Year Book.

Strasburger, Victor. (1992). Children, adolescents and T. V. *Pediatrics in Review, 13*(4), 144–151.

Vaughan, V.C. (1992). Assessment of growth and development during infancy and early childhood. *Pediatrics in Review, 13,* 88–96.

Wasserman, Richard. (1997). Vision Screening. In Robert Hoekelman, ed. *Primary pediatric care* (3rd ed., Ch. 20, pp. 232–234). St. Louis: Mosby–Year Book.

Wells, Robert, & Stein, Martin. (1992). Seven to ten years: The world of the elementary school child. In *Encounters with children: Pediatric behavior and development* (2nd ed., Ch. 23, pp. 329–338). St. Louis: Mosby–Year Book.

Willenger, M., Hoffman, H.J., & Hartford, R.B. (1994). Infant sleep position and risk for sudden infant death syndrome. *Pediatrics, 93,* 814–820.

Wiswell, Thomas. (1995). Neonatal circumcision. *Focus and opinion: Pediatrics, 1*(2), 93–99.

Wolraich, Mark. (1997). Addressing behavioral problems among school-aged children: Traditional and controversial approaches. *Pediatrics in Review, 18*(8), 266–270.

ENDOCRINE AND METABOLIC

Buchanan, George. (1995). Newer concepts in the management of sickle cell disease. *Focus and Opinion: Pediatrics, 1*(2), 100–107.

Chase, H. Peter, & Eisenbarth, George. (1997). Diabetes mellitus. In *Current pediatric diagnosis and treatment* (13th ed., Ch. 30, pp. 857–863). Stamford, CT: Appleton & Lange.

DuPlessis, Helen. (1996). Diabetes mellitus. In Carol Berkowitz, ed. *Pediatrics: A primary care approach* (Ch. 108, pp. 461–465). Philadelphia: Saunders.

Fisher, Delbert. (1994). Hypothyroidism. *Pediatrics in Review, 15*(6), 227–232.

Goodman, Steven, & Greene, Carol. (1994). Metabolic disorders of the newborn. *Pediatrics in Review, 15*(9), 359–365.

Gotlin, Ronald, Kappy, Michael, & Slover, Robert. (1997). Endocrine disorders. In *Current pediatric diagnosis and treatment* (13th ed., Ch. 29, pp. 831–833). Stamford, CT: Appleton & Lange.

Kinney, Thomas, & Ware, Russell. (1988). Advances in the management of sickle cell disease. *Pediatric Consult, 7*(3), 1–7.

Kulin, Howard, & Muller, Jorn. (1996). The biologic aspects of puberty. *Pediatrics in Review, 17*(3), 75–86.

Lane, Peter, Nuss, Rachelle, & Ambruso, Daniel. (1997). Hematologic disorders. In *Current pediatric diagnosis and treatment* (13th ed., Ch. 26, pp. 747–750). Stamford, CT: Appleton & Lange.

Lee, Peter. (1994). Laboratory monitoring of children with precocious puberty. *Archives of Pediatric and Adolescent Medicine, 148,* 369–376.

Mentzer, William. (1996). Sickle cell disease. In *Rudolph's pediatrics* (20th ed., Ch. 17.2.5, pp. 1203–1207). Stamford, CT: Appleton & Lange.

Ogamdi, Simon, & White, George. (1993). Sickle cell disease: Detection and management. *Clinician Reviews,* 65–84.

Oski, Frank, & Johnson, Kevin. (1997). Growth, growth hormone and pituitary disorders. In *Oski's essential pediatrics* (Ch. 176, pp. 482–486). Philadelphia: Lippincott–Raven.

Ott, Mary Jane, & Jackson, Patricia L. (1989). Precocious puberty. Identifying early sexual development. *Nurse Practitioner, 14*(11), 21–30.

Plotnick, Leslie. (1994). Insulin-dependent diabetes mellitus. *Pediatrics in Review, 15*(4), 137–148.

Rosenfeld, Ron. (1996). Growth hormone. *Pediatrics in Review, 17*(4), 143–144.

Sills, Irene. (1994). Hyperthyroidism. *Pediatrics in Review, 15*(11), 417–421.

Zimmerman, D., & Gan-Gaisano, M. (1990). Hyperthyroidism in children and adolescents. *Pediatric Clinics of North America, 37,* 1273–1295.

EYE, EAR, NOSE, AND THROAT

Abbasi, Saify, & Cunningham, Allan. (1996). Are we overtreating sinusitis? *Contemporary Pediatrics, 13*(10), 49–62.

American Academy of Pediatrics. (1994). Managing otitis media with effusion in young children. *Pediatrics, 94*(5), 766–773.

American Academy of Pediatrics. (1995). Treatment of acute streptococcal pharyngitis and prevention of rheumatic fever: A statement for health professionals. *Pediatrics, 96*(4), 758–764.

Berman, Stephen, & Chan, Ken. (1997). Ear, nose and throat. In *Current pediatric diagnosis and treatment* (13th ed., Ch. 17, pp. 416–417). Stamford, CT: Appleton & Lange.

Bodor, Frank, Marchant, Colin, Shurin, Paul, & Barenkamp, Stephen. (1985). Bacterial etiology of conjunctivitis–otitis media syndrome. *Pediatrics, 76*(1), 26–28.

Eisenbaum, Allan. (1997). Eye. In *Current pediatric diagnosis and treatment* 13th ed., Ch. 15, pp. 375–392). Stamford, CT: Appleton & Lange.

Barnett, Elizabeth, and the Greater Boston Otitis Media Study Group. Comparison of ceftriaxone and trimethoprim-sulfamethoxazole for acute otitis media. *Pediatrics, 99*(1), 23–28.

Gigliotti, Francis. (1995). Acute conjunctivitis. *Pediatrics in Review, 16*(6), 203–208.

Hanson, Mary Jane. (1996). Acute otitis media in children. *Nurse Practitioner, 21*(5), 72–80.

Klein, Betty, & Sears, Marvin. (1992). Pediatric ocular injuries. *Pediatrics in Review, 13*(11), 422–428.

Lanphear, Bruce, Auinger, Peggy, Byrd, Robert, & Hall, Caroline. (1997). Increasing prevalence of recurrent otitis media among children in the United States. *Pediatrics, 99*(3), e1 (http://www.pediatrics.org).

Levin, Myron, & Romero, Jose. (1997). Infections: Viral and rickettsial. In *Current pediatric diagnosis and treatment* (13th ed., Ch. 35, pp.980–982). Stamford, CT: Appleton & Lange.

Maxson, Suzanne, & Yamauchi, Terry. (1996). Acute otitis media. *Pediatrics in Review, 17*(6), 191–195.

O'Brien, Rebecca Flynn. (1991). Infectious mononucleosis. *Adolescent Medicine: State of the Art Reviews, 2*(3), 459–471.

Ogle, John. (1997). Infectious bacterial spirochetes. In *Current pediatric diagnosis and treatment* (13th ed., Ch. 37, pp.1017–1020). Stamford, CT: Appleton & Lange.

Pearlman, David, Greos, Leon, & Vitanza, Joanne. (1997) Allergic disorders. In *Current pediatric diagnosis and treatment* (13th ed., Ch. 33, pp. 935–937). Stamford, CT: Appleton & Lange.

Rosenberg, Adam, & Thilo, Elizabeth. (1997). The newborn infant. In *Current pediatric diagnosis and treatment* (13th ed., Ch. 2, pp.22–27). Stamford, CT: Appleton & Lange.

Ruppert, Susan. (1996). Differential diagnosis of common causes of pediatric pharyngitis. *Nurse Practitioner, 21*(4), 38–46.

Stevenson, Linda, & Brooke, Dawn. (1995). Managing otitis media with effusion in young children. *Journal of Pediatric Health Care, 9*(1), 36–39.

Wagner, Rudolph. (1997). Eye infections and abnormalities: Issues for pediatricians. *Contemporary Pediatrics, 14*(6), 137–153.

Wald, Ellen. (1993). Sinusitis. *Pediatrics in Review, 14*(9), 345–350.

Wright, Peter, Thompson, Juliette, & Bess, Fred. (1991). Hearing, speech and language sequelae of otitis media with effusion. *Pediatric Annals, 20*(11), 617–621.

HEMATOLOGIC AND IMMUNOLOGIC

Albano, Edythe, & Pizzo, Philip. (1988). Infectious complications in childhood acute leukemias. *Pediatric Clinics of North America, 35*(4), 873–901.

Albano, Edythe, Stork, Linda, Greffe, Brian, Odom, Lorrie, & Foreman, Nicholas. (1997). Neoplastic disease. In *Current pediatric diagnosis and treatment* (13th ed., Ch. 27, pp. 781–803). Stamford, CT: Appleton & Lange.

American Academy of Pediatrics. (1994). Practice parameter: Management of hyperbilirubinemia in the healthy term newborn. *Pediatrics, 94*, 558.

Avner, Jeffrey. (1997). Occult bacteremia: How great the risk? *Contemporary Pediatrics, 14*(6), 53–65.

Baraff, Larry, Bass, James, Fleisher, Gary, et al. (1993). Practice guidelines for the management of infants and children 0 to 36 months of age with fever without source. *Pediatrics, 12*(1), 1–10.

Bar-on, Miriam, & Boyle, Russell. (1994). Are pediatricians ready for the new guidelines on lead poisoning? *Pediatrics, 93*(2), 178–182.

Bushnell, Francis. (1992). A guide to the primary care of iron deficiency anemia. *Nurse Practitioner, 17*, 68–74.

Bunn, H. Franklin. (1997). Pathogenesis and treatment of sickle cell disease. *The New England Journal of Medicine, 337*(11), 762–769.

Carter, Mary, Thompson, Elizabeth, & Simone, Joseph. (1991). The survivors of childhood solid tumors. *Pediatric Clinics of North America, 38*(2), 505–526.

Centers for Disease Control. (1991). Preventing lead poisoning in young children: A statement by the Centers for Disease Control. Atlanta, Georgia.

Cohen, Bruce, & Garvin, James. (1996). Tumors of the central nervous system. In *Rudolph's pediatrics* (20th ed., Ch. 23.7, pp. 1900–1920). Stamford, CT: Appleton & Lange.

Fletcher, Barry, & Pratt, Charles. (1991). Evaluation of the child with suspected malignant solid tumor. *Pediatric Clinics of North America, 38*(2), 223–248.

Friedman, Henry, Horowitz, Marc, & Oakes, W. Jerry. (1991). Tumors of the central nervous system. *Pediatric Clinics of North America, 38*(2), 381–391.

Gartner, Lawrence. (1994). Neonatal jaundice. *Pediatrics in Review, 15*(11), 422–432.

Kimbrough, Renate, LeVois, Maurice, & Webb, David. (1994). Management of children with slightly elevated blood lead levels. *Pediatrics, 93*(2), 188–191.

Kline, Nancy. (1996). A practical approach to the child with anemia. *Journal of Pediatric Health Care, 10*, 99–105.

Newman, Thomas, & Maisels, M. Jeffrey. (1992). Evaluation and treatment of jaundice in the term newborn: A kinder, gentler approach. *Pediatrics, 89*(5), 809–818.

Oski, Frank. (1992). Hyperbilirubinemia in the term infant: An unjaundiced approach. *Contemporary Pediatrics, 9*(4), 148–154.

Oski, Frank. (1993). Iron deficiency in infancy and childhood. *New England Journal of Medicine, 329*, 190–193.

Oski, Frank. (1997). Fever without localizing signs. In *Oski's Essential pediatrics* (Ch.46). Philadelphia: Lippincott-Raven.

Overby, Kim. (1996). Screening. In *Rudolph's pediatrics* (20th ed., Ch. 1.3, pp. 13–18). Stamford, CT: Appleton & Lange.

Poplack, David, & Reaman, Gregory. (1988). Acute lymphoblastic leukemia in childhood. *Pediatric Clinics of North America, 35*(4), 903–932.

Rosenberg, Adam, & Thilo, Elizabeth. (1997). The newborn infant. In *Current pediatric diagnosis and treatment* (13th ed., Ch. 2, pp. 20–48). Stamford, CT: Appleton & Lange.

Schonfeld, David J., & Needham, Dottie. (1994). Lead: A practical perspective. *Contemporary Pediatrics, 11*, 64–96.

Schwartz, Elias. (1996). Iron deficiency anemia. In R. Behrman, R. Kleigman, & A. Arvin, eds. *Nelson Textbook of pediatrics* (pp. 1387–89). Philadelphia: Saunders.

US Public Health Service. (1994). Put prevention into practice: Lead screening in children. *Journal of the American Academy of Nurse Practitioners, 6*(8), 379–382.

Wheeler, Mark, & Styne, Dennis. (1990). Diagnosis and management of precocious puberty. *Pediatric Clinics of North America, 37*(6), 1255–1269.

Wilson, Debora. (1995). Assessing and managing the febrile child. *Nurse Practitioner, 20*(11), 59–74.

CARDIOVASCULAR

Adams, F.H., Emmanouilides, G.C., & Riemenschneider, T.A. (1989). *Moss' heart disease in infants, children & adolescents* (4th ed.). Baltimore: Williams & Wilkins.

Allen, H.D., Golinko, R.J., & Williams, R.G. (1994). Heart murmurs in children: When is a workup needed? *Contemporary Pediatrics, 11,* 29–52.

Burton, D., & Cabalka, A. (1994). Cardiac evaluation of infants: The first year of life. *Pediatric Clinics of North America, 41*(5), pp. 991–1015.

Fyler, D.C. (1992). *Nadas' pediatric cardiology.* Philadelphia: Hanley & Belfus.

Hazinski, M.F. (1992). *Nursing care of the critically ill child* (2nd ed.). St. Louis: Mosby–Year Book.

McEvoy, M. (1981). Functional heart murmurs. *Nurse Practitioner,* March–April, 34–35.

Robinson, B., Anisman, P., & Eshaghpour, E. (1996). Is that fast heartbeat dangerous?: And what should you do about it. *Contemporary Pediatrics, 13*(9), 52–85.

RESPIRATORY

American Academy of Pediatrics. (1997). Haemophilus influenzae infections. In G. Peter (Ed.), *1997 Red book: Report of the Committee on Infectious Diseases* (24th ed., pp. 220–231). Elk Grove, IL: American Academy of Pediatrics.

American Academy of Pediatrics. (1997). Pertussis. In G. Peter (Ed.), *1997 Red book: Report of the Committee on Infectious Diseases (24th ed.,* pp. 394–407). Elk Grove, IL: American Academy of Pediatrics.

Beeber, S.J. (1996). Parental smoking and childhood asthma. *Journal of Pediatric Health Care, 10*(2), 58–62.

Bell, L.M. (1995). Middle respiratory tract infections: epiglottitis. In H.B. Jenson, & R.S. Baltimore (eds.), *Pediatric infectious diseases: Principles and practice* (pp. 956–959). Stamford, CT: Appleton & Lange.

Centers for Disease Control and Prevention. (1995). Asthma-United States, 1989–1992. *MMWR, 43,* 952–955.

Colizza, D.F. (1995). Pertussis update. *Journal of School Health, 65*(5), 195–198.

Cruz, M.N. (1995). Use of dexamethasone in the outpatient management of acute laryngotracheitis. *Pediatrics, 96,* 220–225.

Fleisher, G.R, & Crain, E.F. (1996). Infectious disease emergencies-croup. In G.R. Fleisher, & S. Ludwig (eds.), *Synopsis of pediatric emergency medicine* (pp. 322–324). Baltimore: Williams & Wilkins.

Fleisher, G.R, & Crain, E.F. (1996). Infectious disease emergencies-epiglottitis. In G.R. Fleisher, & S. Ludwig (eds.), *Synopsis of pediatric emergency medicine* (pp. 323–325). Baltimore: Williams & Wilkins.

Fleisher, G.R, & Crain, E.F. (1996). Infectious disease emergencies-pneumonia. In G.R. Fleisher & S. Ludwig (Eds.), *Synopsis of pediatric emergency medicine* (pp. 326–329). Baltimore: Williams & Wilkins.

Geelhoed, G.C. (1997). Croup. *Pediatric Pulmonology, 23,* 370–374.

Hall, C.B. (1993). Respiratory syncytial virus: What we know now. *Contemporary Pediatrics, 92*–110.

Kemper, K.J. (1997). A practical approach to chronic asthma management. *Contemporary Pediatrics, 14*(8), 86–111.

Klassen, T.P. (1997). Recent advances in the treatment of bronchiolitis and laryngitis. *New Frontiers in Pediatric Drug Therapy, 44*(1), 249–261.

Ladebauche, P. (1997). Managing asthma: A growth and development approach. *Pediatric Nursing, 23*(1), 37–44.

Martinez, F. D., Cline, M., & Barrows, B. (1992). Increased incidence of asthma in children of smoking mothers. *Pediatrics, 89*(1), 21–26.

Martinez, F. D., Wright, A. L., Taussig, L. M., Holberg, C. J., Halonen, M., Morgan, W. J., & the Group Health Medical Associates. (1995). Asthma and wheezing in the first six years of life. *New England Journal of Medicine, 332*(3), 133–138.

National Asthma Education and Prevention Program. (1997). *Expert Panel Report II: Guidelines for the Diagnosis and Management of Asthma.* Bethesda, MD: U.S. Department of Health and Human Services, Publication 97–4051.

Provisional Committee on Quality Improvement. (1994). Practice parameter: The office management of acute exacerbations of asthma in children. *Pediatrics,* 93(1), 119–126.

Rojas, A.R., O'Connell, E.J., & Sachs, M.I. (1991). Chronic cough in children: What to do and why. *The Journal of Respiratory Diseases,* 12(10), 891–903.

Rosenstein, B.J., & Fosarelli, P.D. (1997). Pulmonary diseases. In B.J. Rosenstein, & P.D. Fosarelli, *Pediatric pearls: The handbook of practical pediatrics.* (pp. 315–351). St. Louis: Mosby.

Ruddy, R.M. (1993). Croup—has management changed? *Contemporary Pediatrics.* 21–32.

Ruddy, R.M. (1994). Clearing the air on croup. *Patient Care,* 47–59.

Schidlow, D.V., & Callahan, C.W. (1996). Pneumonia. *Pediatrics In Review,* 17(9), 300–310.

Schwartz, R. (1995). Respiratory syncytial virus in infants and children. *Nurse Practitioner,* 20(9), 24–29.

Toogood, J.H. (1994). Helping your patients make better use of MDI's and spacers. *The Journal of Respiratory Diseases,* 15(2), 151–166.

Urbach, A.H., Bloom, M.D., Mendelsohn, M.J., McIntire, S.C., Gartner, J.C., & Zitelli, B.J. (1993). What's behind that chronic cough? *Contemporary Pediatrics,* 106–127.

Wagner, M.H., & Jacobs, J. (1997). Improving asthma management with peak flow meters. *Contemporary Pediatrics,* 14(8), 111–119.

Welliver, J.R., & Welliver, R.C. (1993). Bronchiolitis. *Pediatrics In Review,* 14(3), 134–139.

Wilmott, R.W. (1997). Cough. In M.W. Schwartz, T.A. Curry, A.J. Sargent, N.J. Blum & J.A. Fein (eds.), *Pediatric primary care: A problem-oriented approach* (3rd ed., pp. 216–224). St. Louis: Mosby.

NEUROLOGIC

Dunn, D.W., & Purvin, V.A. (1990). Headaches in adolescents: Practical management strategies for the pediatrician. *Adolescent Health Update,* 3(1), 1–8.

Goldstein, B., & Powers, K.S. (1994). Head trauma in children. *Pediatrics In Review,* 15(6), 127–131.

Huff, K.R. (1996). Tics. In C.D. Berkowitz, *Pediatrics: A primary care approach,* (pp. 377–380). Philadelphia: W.B. Saunders.

Painter, M.J. & Bergman, I. (1994). Neurology. In R.E. Behrman, & R.M. Kliegman, *Nelson essentials of pediatrics* (2nd ed., pp. 657–708). Philadelphia: W.B. Saunders.

Rosenstein, B.J., & Fosarelli, P.D. (1997). *Pediatric pearls: The handbook of practical pediatrics.* St. Louis: Mosby.

Schutzman, S.A. (1996). Injury-head. In G.R. Fleisher, & S. Ludwig (eds.), *Synopsis of pediatric emergency medicine,* (pp. 596–604). Baltimore: Williams & Wilkins.

Taketomo, C.K., Hodding, J.H., & Kraus, D.M. (1996). *Pediatric dosage handbook.* Cleveland: Lexi-Comp.

Weiss, J. (1993). Assessment and management of the client with headaches. *Nurse Practitioner,* 18(4), 46–57.

GASTROINTESTINAL

American Academy of Pediatrics. (1996). Practice parameter: The management of acute gastroenteritis in young children. *Pediatrics* (97), 424–436.

Buzby, Marianne. (1997). Acute diarrheal illnesses in children. *Lippincott's Primary Care Practice,* 1(3), 252–269.

Cohen, Mitchell B. (1996). Evaluation of the child with acute diarrhea. In *Rudolph's pediatrics* (20th ed., Ch. 15.7.4, pp. 1034–36). Stamford, CT: Appleton & Lange.

Ellett, Marsha. (1990). Constipation/encopresis: A nursing perspective. *Journal of Pediatric Health Care,* 4, 141–146.

Galen, Barbara. (1997). Acute gastroenteritis. *Lippincott's Primary Care Practice,* 1(3), 328–335.

Howe, Allison, & Walker, Eugene. (1992). Behavioral managment of toilet training, enuresis and encopresis. *Pediatric Clinics of North America,* 39(3), 413–432.

Kirschner, Barbara. (1996). Ulcerative colitis in children. *Pediatric Clinics of North America,* 43(1), 235–254.

Kneepkens, C.M., & Hoekstra, J.H. (1996). Chronic nonspecific diarrhea of childhood: Pathophysiology and management. *Pediatric Clinics of North America,* 43(2), 375–390.

Lewis, L. Glen, & Rudolph, Colin. (1997). Practical approach to defecation disorders in children. *Pediatric Annals,* 26(4), 260–268.

Lieberman, J.M. (1994). Rotavirus and other viral causes of gastroenteritis. *Pediatric Annals* (23), 529–535.

Loening-Baucke, Vera. (1996). Encopresis and soiling. *Pediatric Clinics of North America, 43*(1), 279–298.

Milla, Peter J. (1996). Hirschsprung disease and other neuropathies. In *Rudolph's pediatrics* (20th ed., Ch. 15.23.3, pp. 1115–1118). Stamford, CT: Appleton & Lange.

Nolan, Terry, & Oberklaid, Frank. (1993). New concepts in the management of encopresis. *Pediatrics in Review, 14*(11), 447–451.

Oberlander, Tim, & Rappaport, Leonard. (1993). Recurrent abdominal pain during childhood. *Pediatrics in Review, 14*(8), 313–319.

Oski, Frank, & Johnson, Kevin. (1997). Chronic nonspecific diarrhea of childhood. In *Oski's essential pediatrics* (Ch. 155, pp. 427–428). Philadelphia: Lippincott–Raven.

Oski, Frank, & Johnson, Kevin. (1997). Appendicitis. In *Oski's essential pediatrics* (Ch. 167, pp. 454–456). Philadelphia: Lippincott–Raven.

Oski, Frank, & Johnson, Kevin. (1997). Genitourinary disorders. In *Oski's essential pediatrics* (Ch. 138, pp. 385–393). Philadelphia: Lippincott–Raven.

Oski, Frank, & Johnson, Kevin. (1997). Intussusception. In *Oski's essential pediatrics* (Ch. 158, pp. 434–436). Philadelphia: Lippincott–Raven.

Pickering, Larry K. (1996). Salmonella, shigella, and enteric *E. coli* infections. In *Rudolph's pediatrics* (20th ed., Ch. 8.2.21, pp. 592–601). Stamford, CT: Appleton & Lange.

Schmitt, Barton. (1997). Encopresis. In Robert Hoekelman ed. *Primary pediatric care* (3rd ed. Ch. 81, pp. 722–726). St. Louis: Mosby–Year Book.

Stevenson, Richard, & Ziegler, Moritz. (1993). Abdominal pain unrelated to trauma. *Pediatrics in Review, 14*(8), 302–311.

Winesett, Michelle. (1997). Inflammatory bowel disease in children and adolescents. *Pediatric Annals, 26*(4), 227–234.

GENITOURINARY

Andrich, M.P., & Massoud, M. (1992). Diagnostic imaging in the evaluation of the first urinary tract infection in infants and young children. *Pediatrics, 90*, 436–441.

Cronan, K.M. & Norman, M.E. (1995). Renal and electrolyte emergencies. In G.R. Fleisher & S. Ludwig (eds.), *Synopsis of pediatric emergency medicine* (pp. 357–383). Baltimore: Williams & Wilkins.

Heldrich, F.J. (1995). UTI diagnosis: Getting it right the first time. *Contemporary Pediatrics, 12*(2), 110–133.

Langman, C.B. (1993). Proteinuria. In Dershewitz, R.A., *Ambulatory pediatrics* (2nd ed., pp. 449–451). Philadelphia: J.B. Lippincott.

Leonard, M.B., & Shaw, K.N. (1997). Urinary tract infections. In M.W. Schwartz, T.A. Curry, A.J. Sargent, N.J. Blum, & J.A. Fein (eds.), *Pediatric primary care: A problem-oriented approach* (3rd ed., pp. 216–224). St. Louis: Mosby.

Lum, G.M. (1997). Kidney and urinary tract. In W.W. Hay, J.R. Groothuis, A.R. Hayward, & M.J. Levin (Eds.), *Current pediatric diagnosis & treatment* (13th ed., pp. 607–631). Stamford, CT: Appleton & Lange.

Norman, M.E. (1997). Hematuria. In M.W. Schwartz, T.A. Curry, A.J. Sargent, N.J. Blum & J.A. Fein (eds.). *Pediatric primary care: A problem-oriented approach (3rd ed.,* pp. 275–279). St. Louis: Mosby.

Tarry, W. (1997). Urology. In M.W. Schwartz, T.A. Curry, A.J. Sargent, N.J. Blum, & J.A. Fein (eds.), *Pediatric primary care: A problem-oriented approach* (3rd ed., pp. 711–712). St. Louis: Mosby.

Todd, J.K. (1995). Management of urinary tract infections: Children are different. *Pediatrics In Review, 16*(5), 190–196.

GYNECOLOGIC

Beck, W. (1993). *Obstetrics and gynecology* (3rd ed., pp. 11–13). Media, PA: Harwal Publishing.

Campbell, J., & Humphreys, J. (1993). *Nursing care of abused women in nursing care of survivors of family violence* (pp. 248–289). St. Louis: Mosby–Year Book.

Emans, S.J., & Goldstein, D.P. (1990). *Pediatric and adolescent gynecology* (3rd ed., pp. 56, 67–80, 284–286). Boston: Little, Brown.

Frederickson, H., & Wilkins-Haug, L. (1991). *Ob/Gyn Secrets* (pp. 1, 82–85, 135). St. Louis: Mosby–Year Book.

Gerchufsky, M. (1996). Human papilloma virus. *Advance for Nurse Practitioners,* May, 21–26.

Hawkins, J., Roberto, D., Stanley-Haney, J.L. (1993). *Protocols for nurse practitioners in gynecologic settings* (pp. 75–77, 118–199, 139–142, 165–168, 168–171). New York: The Tiresias Press.

Kerouac, S., Taggart, M.E., Lescop, J., Fortin, M.E. (1986). Dimensions of health in violent families. *Health Care for Women International, 7,* 413–426.

Lewis-O'Connor, Annie. (1997). *Family Violence Resource Manual: A Primary Health Care Provider's Guide to Family Violence.* Published by Neighborhood Health Plan. A manual of 250 pages on family violence.

Lewis-O'Connor, A. (1995). Interviewing strategies for special situations. In L. Sims, D. D' Amico, J. Stiesmeyer, & J. Webster, eds. *Health assessment in nursing* (pp. 723–726). Reading, MA: Addison-Wesley.

Lichtman, R., & Papera, S. (1990). *Gynecology well women care* (pp. 51–52, 223–227, 453–454). Norwalk, CT: Appleton & Lange.

Neinstein, L.S. (1984). *Adolescent health care—A practical guide* (pp. 393, 480, 522). Baltimore: Urban & Schwarzenberg.

Ricchini, W. (1997). Break the silence—Talking to your patients about STD's. *Advance for Nurse Practitioners,* June, 55, 56, 83.

Star, W., Lommel, L., & Shannon, M. (1995). Women's Primary Health Care—Protocols for Practice. Published by the American Nurses Association. Washington D.C. Sections 7.3, 12–18, 13–3, 13–10, 13–26, 13–30.

DERMATOLOGIC

American Academy of Pediatrics. (1997). Kawasaki Disease. In G. Peter, ed. *1997 Red book: Report of the Committee on Infectious Diseases* (24th ed., pp. 316–319). Elk Grove Village, IL: American Academy of Pediatrics.

Berkowitz, Carol. (1996). Papulosquamous eruptions. In *Pediatrics: A primary care approach* (Ch. 92, pp. 392–400). Philadelphia: Saunders.

Bisno, Alan, & Stevens, Dennis. (1996). Streptococcal infections of skin and soft tissues. *The New England Journal of Medicine, 334*(4), 240–245.

Buckley, Rebecca. (1996). Urticaria and angioedema. In *Rudolph's Pediatrics* (20th ed., Ch. 7.4.8, pp. 473–474). Stamford, CT: Appleton & Lange.

Ceballos, Patricia, Ruiz-Maldonado, Ramon, & Mihm, Martin. (1995). Melanoma in children. *The New England Journal of Medicine, 332*(10), 656–662.

Cohen, Bernard. (1992). Atopic dermatitis: Breaking the itch–scratch cycle. *Contemporary Pediatrics, 6,* 64–81.

Cohen, Bernard. (1993). *Atlas of pediatric dermatology.* London: Mosby–Wolfe.

Cohen, Bernard. (1997). Warts and children: Can they be separated? *Contemporary Pediatrics, 14*(2), 128–149.

Frieden, Ilona. (1996). Infections and infestations. In *Rudolph's Pediatrics* (20th ed., Ch. 12.13, pp. 929–938). Stamford, CT: Appleton & Lange.

Frieden, Ilona, & Resnick, Steven. (1991). Childhood exanthems: Old and new. *Pediatric Clinics of North America, 38*(4), 859–882.

Halbert, Anne. (1996). The practical management of atopic dermatitis in children. *Pediatric Annals, 25*(2), 72–28.

Healy, Eugene, & Simpson, Nick. (1994). Acne vulgaris. *British Medical Journal, 308,* 831–833.

Hebert, Adelaide, & Goller, Michelle. (1996). Papulosquamous disorders in the pediatric patient. *Contemporary Pediatrics, 13*(2), 69–88.

Heyman, Peter, Rakes, Gary, Loach, Thomas, & Murphy, Deborah. (1997). Recognizing the young atopic child. *Contemporary Pediatrics, 14*(4), 131–39.

Honig, P. (1986). Arthropod bites, stings and infestations: Their prevention and treatment. *Pediatric Dermatology, 3,* 189–197.

Hurwitz, Sidney. (1994). Acne vulgaris: Pathogenesis and management. *Pediatrics in Review, 15*(2), 47–52.

Krowchuk, Daniel, Tunnessen, Walter, & Hurwitz, Sidney. (1992). Pediatric dermatology update. *Pediatrics, 90*(2), 259–264.

Morelli, Joseph, & Weston, William. (1997) Skin. In *Current pediatric diagnosis and treatment* (13th ed., Ch. 14, pp. 357–374). Stamford, CT: Appleton & Lange.

Pattishall, Evan III. (1997). Chickenpox. In Robert Hoekelman, ed. *Primary pediatric care* (3rd ed., Ch. 191, pp. 1239–1243). St. Louis: Mosby–Year Book.

Pearlman, David, Greos, Leon, & Vitanza, Joanne. (1997). Allergic disorders. In *Current pediatric diagnosis and treatment* (13th ed., Ch. 33, pp. 922–943). Stamford, CT: Appleton & Lange.

Prose, Neil. (1996). Acne and related disorders. In *Rudolph's pediatrics* (20th ed., Ch. 12.10.4, pp. 924–925). Stamford, CT: Appleton & Lange.

Prose, Neil. (1996). Other papulosquamous disorders. In *Rudolph's pediatrics* (20th ed., Ch. 12.3.5, pp. 894–895). Stamford, CT: Appleton & Lange.

Schiff, Richard. (1996). Anaphylaxis. In *Rudolph's pediatrics* (20th ed., Ch. 7.4.9, pp. 474–475). Stamford, CT: Appleton & Lange.

Sifuentes, Monica. (1996). Dermatologic disorders: Acne. In *Pediatrics: A primary care approach.* (Ch. 89, pp. 381–384). Philadelphia: Saunders.

Vasiloudes, Panos, Morelli, Joseph, & Weston, William. (1997). A guide to rashes in newborns. *Contemporary Pediatrics, 14*(6), 156–166.

Weinberg, Adriana, & Levin, Myron. (1997). Infections: Parasitic and mycotic. In *Current pediatric diagnosis and treatment* (13th ed., Ch. 38, pp. 1061–1094). Stamford, CT: Appleton & Lange.

Williams, Larry. (1996). Atopic dermatitis. In *Rudolph's Pediatrics* (20th ed., Ch. 7.4.7, pp. 769–73). Stamford, CT: Appleton & Lange.

MUSCULOSKELETAL

Aronsson, D., Goldberg, M., Kling, T., & Roy, D. (1994). Developmental dysplasia of the hip. *Pediatrics, 94*(2), 201–208.

Brady, M. (1993). The child with a limp. *The Journal of Pediatric Health Care, 7*(5), 226–228.

Conrad, E.U. (1989). Pitfalls in diagnosis: Pediatric musculoskeletal tumors. *Pediatric Annals, 18*(1), 45–52.

Craig, C., & Goldberg, M. (1993). Foot and leg problems. *Pediatrics in Review, 14*(10), 395–400.

Grogan, D.P., & Ogden, J.A. Knee and ankle injuries in children. *Pediatrics in Review, 13*(11), 429–434.

Jackman, K.V. (1994). Acute pediatric orthopedic conditions. *Pediatric Annals, 23*, 240–249.

Novacheck, T. (1996). Developmental dysplasia of the hip. *Pediatric Clinics of North America, 43*(4), 829–847.

Renshaw, T. (1995). The child who has a limp. *Pediatrics in Review, 16*(12), 458–465.

Rudy, C. (1996). Developmental dysplasia of the hip: What's new in the 90's? *The Journal of Pediatric Health Care, 10*(2), 85.

Sponseller, P.D. (1997). Orthopedics. In B.J. Rosenstein, & P.D. Fosarelli, *Pediatric pearls: The handbook of practical pediatrics* (pp.259–262). St. Louis: Mosby.

Tachdjian, M.O. (1997). *Clinical pediatric orthopedics: The art of diagnosis and principles of management.* Stamford, CT: Appleton & Lange.

Tolo, V., & Wood, B. (1993). *Pediatric orthopedics in primary care.* Baltimore: Williams & Wilkins.

INFECTIOUS DISEASES

American Academy of Pediatrics. (1997). Lyme disease. In G. Peter (ed.), *1997 Red book: Report of the Committee on Infectious Diseases* (24th ed., pp. 329–333). Elk Grove, IL: American Academy of Pediatrics.

American Academy of Pediatrics. (1997). Tuberculosis. In G. Peter (ed.), *1997 Red book: Report of the Committee on Infectious Diseases* (24th ed., pp. 541–562). Elk Grove, IL: American Academy of Pediatrics.

Berti, L.C. (1997). Childhood tuberculosis. *The Journal of Pediatric Health Care, 10*(3), 131–134.

Committee On Infectious Disease (American Academy of Pediatrics). (1994). Screening for tuberculosis in infants and children. *Pediatrics, 93*(1), 131–134.

Jacobs, R.F., & Starke, J.R. (1993). Tuberculosis in children. *Medical Clinics of North America, 77*(6), 1335–1351.

Jenson, H.B., & Baltimore, R.S. (1995). *Pediatric infectious diseases: Principles and practices.* Stamford, CT: Appleton & Lange.

Moskowitz, H., & Meissner, H.C. (1997). Tick-borne diseases: Warm weather worry. *Contemporary Pediatrics, 14*(8), 33–49.

Rowley, A.H., & Shulman, S.T. (1995). Kawasaki syndrome. In H.B. Jenson, & R.S. Baltimore, *Pediatric infectious diseases: Principles and practice* (pp. 629–638). Stamford, CT: Appleton & Lange.

GENETIC ISSUES

American Academy of Pediatrics. (1995). Committee on Genetics: Health supervision for children with Turner syndrome. *Pediatrics, 96*(6), 1166–1172.

American Academy of Pediatrics. (1996). Committee on Genetics: Health supervision for children with fragile X syndrome. *Pediatrics, 98*(2), 297–300.

Carey, John. (1992). Health supervision and anticipatory guidance for children with genetic disorders. *Pediatric Clinics of North America, 39*(1), 25–53.

Castiglia, Patricia. (1997). Turner syndrome. *The Journal of Pediatric Health Care, 11*(1), 34–36.

Sujansky, Eva, Stewart, Janet, & Manchester, David. (1997). Genetics and dysmorphology. In *Current pediatric diagnosis and treatment* (13th ed., Ch. 32, pp. 894–895). Stamford, CT: Appleton & Lange.

MISCELLANEOUS DISEASES AND DISORDERS

American Psychiatric Association. (1994). *Diagnostic and statistical manual of mental disorders (4th ed.).* Washington, D.C.

Baren, M. (1994). ADHD: Do we finally have it right? *Contemporary Pediatrics, 11,* 96–124.

Baren, M. (1994). Managing ADHD. *Contemporary Pediatrics, 11,* 29–48.

Bithoney, W.G., Dubowitz, H., & Egan, H. (1992). Failure to thrive/Growth deficiency. *Pediatrics in Review, 13*(12), 453–460.

Borowsky, I.W. (1996). Attention deficit hyperactivity disorder. In Carol Berkowitz. *Pediatrics: A primary care approach* (pp. 404–407). Philadelphia: W.B. Saunders.

Burns, C.E. & Shelton, K.C. (1996). Cognitive-Perceptual Patterns. In: C.E. Burns, N. Barber, M.A. Brady, & A.M. Dunn, *Pediatric primary care: A handbook for nurse practitioners.* Philadelphia: W.B. Saunders.

Frank, D.A., Silva, M., & Needlman, R. (1993). Failure to thrive: Mystery, myth, and method. *Contemporary Pediatrics,* 114–133.

Meghdadpour, S. (1997). Cystic fibrosis. In J.A. Fox (Ed.), *Primary Health Care of Children* (pp. 849–858). St. Louis: Mosby.

TRAUMA AND EMERGENCIES

Berkowitz, C. (1996). Physical abuse. In Carol Berkowitz, (ed.), *Pediatrics: A primary care approach* (pp. 408–411). Philadelphia: W.B. Saunders.

Davis, H.W., & Zitelli, B.J. (1995). Childhood injuries: Accidental or inflicted? *Contemporary Pediatrics,* (12), 94–112.

Fleisher, G.R., & Ludwig, S. (1996). *Synopsis of pediatric emergency medicine.* Baltimore: Williams & Wilkins.

Hendretig, F., & Shannon, M. (1996). Toxicologic Emergencies. In G.R. Fleisher & S. Ludwig (eds.), *Synopsis of pediatric emergency medicine* (pp. 447–462). Baltimore: Williams & Wilkins.

Lease, J.G. (1992). Office care of wounds. *Pediatrics in Review, 13*(7), 257–261.

Rosenstein, B.J., & Fosarelli, P.D. (1997). *Pediatric pearls: The handbook of practical pediatrics.* St. Louis: Mosby.

PROFESSIONAL ISSUES

American Academy of Nurse Practitioners. (1993). *Standards of practice.* Washington, DC: American Academy of Nurse Practitioners.

ANA. (1987). *Standards of practice for the primary health care nurse practitioner.* Washington, DC: ANA.

Congressional Budget Office, US Congress. (April 1989). *Physician extenders: Their current and future role in medical care delivery.* Washington, DC: US Government Printing Office.

Jacox, Ada. (1989). The OTA Report: A policy analysis. *Nursing Outlook, 35,* 262–267.

Kulal, Stephanie, & Clever, Linda. (1994). Acceptance of the nurse practitioner. *American Journal of Nursing,* pp. 251–256.

Pearson, Linda J. (Jan. 1993). 1992–1993 Update: How each state stands on legislative issues affecting advanced nursing practice. *Nurse Practitioner, 18,* 23–38.

Prescott, P.A., & Driscoll, L. (1990). Evaluating nurse practitioner performance. *Nurse Practitioner, 25,* 28–32.

Record, J.C., ed. (1990). Provided requirements, cost savings and the new health practitioner in primary care: National estimate for 1996, Contract 231-77-0077. Washington, DC: DEHEW.

Smith, K.R. (1995). Health practitioners: Efficient utilization and cost of health care. *Journal of Health, Policy and Law, 5,* 451.

Index

Page numbers followed by f and t indicate figures and tables, respectively.